MW00465891

SUGAR
LESS

Also by Nicole M. Avena, PhD

Why Diets Fail: Because You're Addicted to Sugar

What to Eat When You're Pregnant:
A Week-by-Week Guide to Support Your
Health and Your Baby's Development

What to Feed Your Baby and Toddler:
A Month-by-Month Guide to Support
our Child's Health and Development

What to Eat When You Want to Get Pregnant:
A Science-Based 4-Week Nutrition
Program to Boost Your Fertility

A 7-Step Plan to Uncover Hidden Sugars,
Curb Your Cravings, and Conquer Your Addiction

SUGAR LESS

Nicole M. Avena, PhD

Foreword by Daniel Amen, MD

UNION
SQUARE
& CO.

NEW YORK

UNION SQUARE & CO.

NEW YORK

ISBN 978-1-4549-4780-6
ISBN 978-1-4549-4781-3 (e-book)

Library of Congress Control Number: 2023022818
Library of Congress Cataloging-in-Publication Data is available upon request.

For information about custom editions, special sales, and premium
purchases, please contact specialsales@unionsquareandco.com.

Printed in the United States of America

2 4 6 8 10 9 7 5 3 1

unionsquareandco.com

Cover design by Jo Obarowski
Cover photograph by Sarah Jun, © 2023 Union Square & Co., LLC
Interior design by Christine A. Heun
Author photo © 2023 Sameer Khan
Image credits: Creative Market: Bdemm Studio: 4, 56 (label);
Getty Images: DigitalVision Vectors/-VICTOR-: 4, 168, 169, 170, 171;
Shutterstock.com: HIRO-Lab: 8

To Bart

CONTENTS

FOREWORD
BY DANIEL AMEN, MD

I hate sugar. It is a drug that, like other drugs of abuse, hurts your brain. So, when my friend and colleague Dr. Nicole Avena asked me to write the foreword for this book, I was thrilled to do it.

I am a psychiatrist and a brain health expert, and I have devoted my career to helping people of all ages achieve better brain health. Dr. Avena's work on sugar addiction has informed not only my work with patients but also the treatment plans I suggest. Throughout my career, I have come to witness firsthand the negative impact sugar can have on one's overall and brain health. I have seen people struggle with their addiction to sugar, and the damage it has caused to their brains, their relationships, and their bodies. I have also seen the personal struggle that my patients have encountered, and after realizing how bad sugar is for them, the feeling of powerlessness when they can't give it up due to the intense cravings that they encounter. Sugar cravings are a battle between one's inner child, who craves sugar, and the prefrontal cortex, which knows what is best for our health. Throughout the day, your inner child may encourage you to have the doughnut, to include the white bread as a side, and to treat yourself to dessert. Your prefrontal cortex begs you to stop eating sweets, to put down the unneeded carbohydrates, and to consume something with vitamins and minerals. This battle continues day after day, week after week, month after month, and year after year. Often, your inner child wins, cheering you on as you choose the sweet over the vegetable. However, over time, this choice damages your mind and body. Before long, lifestyle conditions such as obesity, diabetes, hypertension, ADHD, and depression are present. To improve the health of your brain and body, this internal battle must stop. For this to happen, reducing one's sugar intake is essential.

Dr. Avena has known all of this for years. In fact, over twenty years ago, when she was a graduate student at Princeton, she conducted the seminal, groundbreaking experiments showing the scientific community that sugar, in fact, is an addictive substance. Do you remember hearing about the rat study where the animals preferred sugar over cocaine? That came from her research! For her PhD dissertation, Nicole developed an animal model of sugar addiction, and systematically tested the American Psychiatric Association's (APA) criteria for substance use disorder, to see whether these criteria could be found when the substance of abuse is sugar. Guess what? Sugar checked *all* the boxes as an addictive substance.

But back then, Nicole's research wasn't immediately well received. It was dubbed "controversial," because no one had scientifically shown that a food and drugs could be classified as equally addictive. Also, people who were struggling to lose weight or who were obese were thought to just not have the "willpower" to control themselves. I knew back then about the addictive hold that sugar had on some of my patients, and thanks to Nicole's early work in this area, most other doctors and scientists are now in agreement with us: sugar is a deadly drug, and it is slowly killing us. It is time to do something about it.

Sugarless has come to the rescue! It reviews the latest science behind sugar addiction and offers readers a way out of the addiction trap. And Nicole is the perfect person to write this book. Not only does she know the science of sugar addiction better than anyone, but with a PhD in neuroscience and psychology, she also knows the practical steps you need to take to help the brain heal. The brain is beautiful and malleable, meaning that YOU can change your brain! You can retrain your brain to beat your addiction to sugar, and in the process reap all the health benefits that come along with it. *Sugarless* is your guide.

However, we know that eating healthfully is easier said than done. *Sugarless* helps readers to see through the marketing traps that food companies use to convince us that processed foods that are high in sugar are fine to eat. They use terms like *all-natural* and *organic* to try to fool us into thinking something is healthy. Also, *Sugarless* helps you in many other ways, including how to deal with sugar withdrawal, how to manage sugar cravings, what to eat to stabilize blood sugar, and so on. By incorporating these tips into your diet, you can reduce your sugar intake to improve your mental and physical health.

I have seen the positive effects that removing sugar can have on one's health and well-being countless times. At the Amen Clinics, we use an integrative approach to diagnosing our patients, including their biological, psychological, social, and spiritual well-being. We use brain imaging, comparing the activity of a patient to a healthy model, to diagnose our patients and create treatment plans. We utilize a functional medicine approach, which includes changes in diet and lifestyle interventions, to heal the brain. I have seen overwhelming success in my patients using this approach, and cutting back on added sugars is key to achieving optimal wellness.

I am so glad that Nicole wrote this book. So many people are struggling with addiction to sugar and want to break free but can't. *Sugarless* is the way out. Nicole breaks down why a low-sugar diet is important and gives readers practical tips on how individuals can achieve this goal. *Sugarless* will help you see the science behind why your previous diets have failed, how quick fixes are unsuccessful, and how you can get on the path of health by ditching the sugar.

INTRODUCTION

In the summer of 2001, most of my friends, like me, had just graduated from college. They had chosen to move to big cities, get fancy jobs, and spend their nights hanging out with friends and going to concerts—typical stuff for twenty-something-year-olds. I, on the other hand, had chosen a different way to spend my evenings. I spent them feeding rats.

Let me back up for a minute and give you some context. I had started graduate school at Princeton University that summer. I arrived in Princeton with a huge case of imposter syndrome. *Imposter syndrome* is the psychological term used to describe the feelings that people can get when they think they don't deserve to be someplace, and that at any moment someone is going to discover they are a fraud or an "imposter" and expose them. (A topic for another book, I suppose.) No one in my family had ever even been to college, and here I was getting a PhD in neuroscience from an Ivy League school. I couldn't help but feel that clearly, someone had made a mistake in letting me in.

Despite the negative voices in my head, I resolved to push forward and do my best. I was assigned to work with a professor named Dr. Bartley Hoebel. His friends and students all called him

Bart. He was a very tall (6'7"-ish), lean man, who had a quiet, gentle nature. He was a true Ivy Leaguer, having trained at the University of Pennsylvania and Harvard, and was now a well-respected professor at Princeton. He was accomplished, with hundreds of published scientific papers on what happens in the brain in response to people engaging in motivated behaviors, like eating, drinking, using drugs, or mating. He was regularly invited to give presentations all over the world to discuss his latest research findings. I thought that his research was fascinating and felt very fortunate to be his student.

One day that summer, Bart asked me to come to his office so that we could have a meeting to talk about what I might want to work on as a research project that I could eventually turn into a PhD dissertation. This had to be a big idea—something that I would work on for the next five years of my life. Little did I know I would still be working on it over twenty years later.

We started to talk about how there was a lot of interest in the scientific community regarding obesity at the time, as there still is now, and media reports often mentioned rising obesity rates. Keep in mind that the year 2001 was a while ago, and back then most people (including doctors) viewed obesity as being caused by a lack of willpower on the part of the individual, and essentially put all the blame on the person who was overweight or obese for being that way.

We began thinking about how it was strange that, despite all the public health warnings concerning the dangers of being obese, and the multimillion-dollar diet industry that offered an array of choices and plans to follow to lose weight, people still couldn't do it. The South Beach Diet®, the Zone Diet®, WeightWatchers®, the Master Cleanse®—these are just a few of the more popular options that many people tried and failed. They were being handed a plan, but it was impossible to stick to. Why? Could it all be about lack of willpower? And if, for argument's sake, it was, what was causing people *not* to have the willpower to make healthier choices about what they ate? For some individuals who had obesity-related comorbid conditions, like diabetes or heart disease, this was a matter of life and death. It seemed like more than willpower was at play here. What if being overweight or obese had less to do with the person and their supposed lack of willpower, and more to do with *what* they were eating?

Thanks to advancements in technology and agriculture, our food supply has continued to evolve. This is a good thing, as it has allowed us to avoid starvation and feed the increasing number of humans that inhabit the earth. However, when we look at the changes that have occurred over the past fifty years, it seems that many of these changes are for the worse. More and more people are relying on fast food, processed grocery store foods, and vending machines as a staple in their diet. And there is a common thread among these foods: they all contain added sugar.

Pour on the Sugar

Sugar. It has been around for centuries, and for most of that time we have lived in harmony with it, but that suddenly is changing. I will get into this more in the next chapter, but back in the early 2000s, we were coming off the "low fat" diet trend that had begun in the 1970s. Fat had been demonized by the American Medical Association (AMA) and other important medical groups because of its supposed negative impact on heart health, and these groups also argued that it caused obesity. To break it down to sound bites for the media: If you eat fat, you will get fat. Fat = bad, carbs = good.

What started this idea? Back in the 1960s a physiologist named Ancel Keys published a theory that dietary fat raises cholesterol levels and gives you heart disease. This began a decades-long era in which *all* dietary fats were thought to be bad for your health. In the late 1970s, "Dietary Goals for the United States" was published, advising Americans to significantly curb their fat intake, and in 1984, the National Institutes of Health (NIH) officially recommended that all Americans over the age of two eat less fat. Turns out, they were all very wrong. But at the time, because the public had been sternly warned to avoid fats in fear that they would die from a heart attack or end up obese, most Americans were ditching the fats and, instead, eating more and more carbohydrates.

This meant that in the 1970s we saw an influx of sugar in our food supply that slowly went up over time. You could see this for yourself when you went to the grocery store. Aisles were lined with "low fat" cookies and snacks, and they all contained added sugars. If you lived through this time period, you may fondly recall SnackWell's®, which were a popular brand of fat-free cookies and other treats.

People were (falsely) led to believe that you could indulge guiltlessly on them, because they were labeled as "fat-free." Back then, it was *fat* that was bad for you, so companies were doing you a favor by taking it out of the products. The problem was that if you take the fat out, the food usually tastes terrible. So the food companies added sugar to make it taste good again. Sugar is a carbohydrate, so it was safe, and heck, better for you than the dreaded fat!

All the while in the background, it was becoming apparent that sugar might not be all that good for us. Sweets were usually—and still are—the main topic of discussion when people wanted to lose weight. Many people for years had been talking about how they craved sugar, had a sweet tooth, and if they were trying to lose weight, giving up the white stuff was the hardest part. Sugar seemed to be a barrier for many people, and it stood in the way of losing weight. Giving up desserts and sweets was usually the tactic to try to lose weight, and usually the downfall for most dieters because it was hard to stick to.

In the latter part of the 1990s another shift occurred. The media had begun to take note of America's inability to give up the white stuff. You could pick up any magazine at the grocery checkout at that time and read a headline about "being hooked on carbs" or "ways to beat your sweet cravings." Mass media hinted that people were hooked, in some way, on sugars and carbohydrates. Were these just sensationalized headlines to grab readers, or was there actually something to this idea?

I started to look more carefully at some of the processed food products that were on the market—many contained so much added sugar, and in amounts that we would never *ever* see in nature. As a neuroscience student, I knew that the parts of the brain that evolved to regulate our appetite were used to concentrations of sugar that were more like what you would find in nature—for example, in an apple. But now, our brains were being blasted multiple times each day with the effects of ten times that amount of sugar from cookies, cakes, and protein bars. Not to mention all the sugar-laden foods that people were eating because they thought they were healthy, like some yogurts, salad dressings, and even fruit smoothies.

It reminded me of what happens with drugs like heroin and cocaine. Part of the reason drugs like these are so addictive is because they over-activate the brain reward centers (more on this in chapter 3). They hijack the reward system and set our pleasure into overdrive. Drugs make you feel good (at first, at least), and our brain adapts accordingly to make us crave that feeling again and again, which makes us do almost anything to get it. I started to ponder: What if these processed foods that were so commonplace in our society, with loads of added sugar, were hijacking our brains in the same ways that drugs of abuse do? Could people be hooked on sugar in the way people get "hooked" on other things, like drugs and alcohol? Could people actually get *addicted* to sugar?

After our initial discussion, Bart asked me to look into the scientific literature to see what I could come up with about sugar addiction as a basis for my dissertation. Excited to prove how great a student I was and to confirm to my inner monologue that Princeton was correct to admit me, I went off to the library to put together a literature review to discuss at our next meeting. But after hours and hours of scouring the medical and science databases for papers looking at sugar addiction, I came up with nothing. Not one single empirical study examined this. The term *sugar addiction* doesn't even appear in search databases until 2002 (when we started publishing about it). Decades of diet and obesity research was out there, and none of it even flirted with using the term *addiction*. If anything, there were numerous studies fueled by the focus on heart health, suggesting that sugar and other carbohydrates were *better* for you than fat-rich foods.

I felt deflated. One of the first things they teach you in graduate school is that when doing research, you need to have some literature (i.e., a strong basis) to back up your idea. You can't just pull an idea out of the sky and do a dissertation on it! Now, the imposter syndrome was really kicking in. I would have to go back and tell Bart that I couldn't find anything to support this idea, and I would have to slink back to the drawing board and come up with something else to study. But the next day, when I met with him and I told him about my failed search, he said something that completely changed my life. Instead of sending me off to come up with another topic to study, which is what I was expecting, he said, "I have a feeling this is something big. And if there are no studies on this, you better get down to the lab and start doing them."

It's 10 p.m., Time to Feed the Rats

Since we were starting from scratch with this idea, we had to come up with a model to test it. Bart had a rat lab, which was fortunate because looking back, it would have been impossible to do any of our initial studies on people, since finding participants to be in the control group that never tasted sugar would have been a challenge! So we developed a rat model where we allowed rats twelve hours each day to drink sugar, and then took it away (I'll tell you more about the rats and the model in chapter 3). The idea of sugar addiction was completely new, so we didn't have a big grant or much money at all in the budget to support these initial studies. That meant we had to be creative and industrious. Every night, one of my lab mates or I would go into the lab at 10 p.m. and take sugar away from the rats. My boyfriend (who was crazy enough to date someone with this type of work schedule and is now my husband) and friends all got used to me abruptly leaving the DBar, the shabby yet cozy on-campus bar and general hangout place for graduate students at Princeton, when I needed to go measure how much sugar the rats were drinking. Looking back, it was rather strange to leave my friends to go feed rats while they ordered another round of drinks, but at the time it felt completely normal.

I won't go into what happens next in the research, because you'll read about all of that in chapter 3. But I will tell you that we set out conducting a series of experiments to try to answer the question: Is sugar addictive? Twenty-two years later, together with my lab colleagues, I have published over a hundred scholarly research papers on this topic. And we aren't the only ones. Many, many more researchers have become interested in the effects that sugar has on our health, and there are now *thousands* of research papers on the topic of sugar and how too much of it can be dangerous to our health. The tide has dramatically changed, and sugar addiction is well established as a contributing factor to obesity, overeating, and poor health in general.

What's Next?

That is the story of how I got here. Now, let me tell you why I stayed here.

I have learned so much over my career about the damaging effects of sugar, and the damage goes even further than I initially thought. Sugar has not only been shown to have destructive effects on metabolic health, but new research shows that it can negatively impact learning, memory, impulse control, and metabolism as well, just to name a few things. Many of the medical conditions that plague adults, such as diabetes, cardiovascular disease, and fatty liver disease, are now being tied back to our diet—with sugar as the main culprit.

Sugar is a silent killer. The damage that sugar causes isn't obvious at first, and there aren't always outward signs that anything bad is happening to your brain or body because of having too much of it. You aren't going to drop dead from eating one cookie, but many years of having a poor diet that is rich in added sugar will not only reduce your life span, but it will also make it much more likely to be fraught with illness, disease, and unhappiness.

The worst part about all of it is that, despite the fact that we *know* all of this, we continue to live in a world that is sugar-centric. Sugar is everywhere. It is pushed on our kids from a young age. It's at the checkout line in almost every store. It is hidden in food products using different names. It is unavoidable. And if you happen to be one of the many people whose brain has been hijacked by it, you are stuck in the sugar vortex and probably feel like you can't get out.

Most people move on from their PhD dissertation and end up studying something else. I often tell people that, even though Princeton gave me my PhD degree almost twenty years ago, and my imposter syndrome has mostly cured itself, I am still working on my dissertation. There is so much more work to do. While I am still doing research, my focus has shifted toward helping people to *understand* the research, and to *use it* to their advantage. That is why I wrote this book.

I have been inspired by the stories that people have shared with me of both anguish and success, and I want to help. I want to help you break free from your sugar addiction. I want you to have first-degree access to the science so you can understand what sugar does to your brain, and how it can grab hold of your ability to control your intake. But more importantly, I want to empower you with the psychological and behavioral skills and tools that you need to break from the powerful hold of sugar and change your brain in a way that will change your life, forever.

How This Book Can Help

This isn't a diet book. The last thing anyone needs is another diet book.

This book is different because it's a *science* and *psychology* book.

The science is key to making logical sense of what you should and shouldn't eat. I will talk about the studies, so for example, when you have a craving for sweets, you can remember that the hedonically programmed part of your brain is causing you to have that craving, not the actual need for food! The goal is to help you see that sugar is the culprit behind your overeating, your weight gain, and your unhappiness. Sugar not only messes up your metabolic health, but it also messes with your brain. By changing the way your neurons communicate, sugar traps you further into a spiral of addiction: bingeing, withdrawal, and craving. I will get into the neuroscience and the studies about this in chapter 3, but for now, know that sugar addiction is real, and it is screwing up your brain.

But don't worry—I can help you fix this. In chapter 1, I will review how sugar can lead to overeating, how our diet culture has damaged us, and how sugar has been linked to obesity and other mental and physical health conditions. Then, in chapter 2, I'll review the latest research on the influx of sugar in the American diet, and discuss sources of sugar that people may not even be aware of (guess what? Your bacon has sugar in it! And so do your English muffins). This chapter will show you how easy it is to overeat sugar, even when you may *think* you are eating a low-sugar diet and making healthy choices. Next, in chapter 3, I'll review the research on sugar addiction, beginning with my initial studies, and also the latest findings. I'll explain how sugar can impact the brain in ways that drugs such as heroin or cocaine do.

Then, in chapter 4, the real work begins. We'll start to implement the steps to break your addiction to sugar. This chapter will lay out the Seven Simple Steps that readers can use to break their addiction to sugar and achieve sugar freedom. It will describe the steps, how to apply them, and how long each will take. After we assess the severity of your addiction to sugar, I will then help you to change your diet in a structured, simple way. The emphasis here is *replace, don't remove.* I will show you how to systematically replace foods that you love with healthier alternatives so that you won't feel deprived. The goal is for you to change your mindset completely around diets and food—you will not be "on a diet." Instead, this is a new way of healthier eating that will be soon become your new happy norm.

The next chapter is important because it will help you navigate common hurdles that people face when they give up sugars. In chapter 5, I will talk about some common foods that can help to make giving up sugar easier, including my ten Craving Crushing Foods—high-fiber foods to help regulate blood sugar and higher protein foods to help reduce cravings. Also, I'll discuss triggers, and how to handle them. Then, I will review the research on sugar withdrawal and cravings and offer practical tips on how to manage these inevitable components of kicking a sugar addiction. Just like people who get addicted to drugs and alcohol experience withdrawal when they give them up, the same can happen with sugar. I'll review how to cope with withdrawal and offer a timeline on what to expect. Cravings are a natural part of being human, but most people don't know whether a craving is biological (i.e., we have low blood sugar, or low iron, and our body is physiologically in need of food), or something else. I will teach you about "hedonic cravings," which are just cravings for the pleasure we get from eating foods, and how these are typically why we crave sweets. Don't worry—I will also teach you how to survive them without giving in!

Then in chapter 6, I will talk about how to live your new life, managing what I call the three S's that are key to your success. These are: stressors, setbacks, and social pressures around food. Not knowing how to deal with these S's will put you in a position that can lead you to relapse and go back to your old ways of eating. I will discuss the food environment and how we are essentially fighting an uphill battle to avoid sugar, thanks to the media, the food industry, and our own daily routines. This chapter will talk about relapses and provide psychological insights into why they occur, how you can avoid them, and what you can do if one happens so that you don't feel you have failed and should just throw in the towel. This chapter will also describe some ways in which you can navigate social situations that involve food that can sometimes become awkward or pressure-packed.

Are you ready? Let's get started!

CHAPTER 1

HOW SUGAR CAUSES YOU TO OVEREAT AND HARMS YOUR HEALTH

You were born to be a sugar addict. It is in your genes.

But don't go cursing your great-great-great-grandparents for making you this way just yet. There's a little more to it, and it starts with basic human anthropology.

We humans evolved to, slowly but surely, adapt to our environment, and what we eat is a *big* part of that environment. Our hunter-and-gatherer ancestors, who foraged in the wilderness for food, quickly learned to equate sweet taste with safety. For example, if our ancestors stumbled across a berry bush, the sweet berries on the bush were safe to eat, but if they ate the rotten, sour ones that had fallen to the forest floor, they likely would get sick, and possibly die. Since the goal was to avoid things that would kill off our species, humans came to develop an innate preference for things that taste sweet.

This sweet preference has served us well, to some extent. The sugar-loving mentality that we inherited helps ensure that infants like breastmilk, which is sweet. This preference for sweet taste also helps humans of all ages enjoy the taste of fruits, which naturally contain sugars along with many important nutrients, and avoid the taste of bitter things that might be spoiled or contain toxins. In fact, our acceptance nowadays to eat somewhat bitter foods because of their known health benefits (like broccoli) is somewhat forced—our genes tell us not to, but the rational part of the brain wins out because we know they are safe and healthy. But something has changed in our environment that turned our love for sugar from being a survival mechanism into something that is slowly killing us.

The Evolution of Food

A lot of things have changed since our ancestor hunters and gatherers roamed the earth. Now, we modern-day hunters and gatherers still forage for food, but in a very different environment. For one, we don't have to work very hard to get food. We can click a button online and get groceries delivered. No need to wander around all day looking for some edible grasses; Uber Eats® will deliver!

Second, the menu has changed. We no longer have a finite and very limited number of options for nourishment, which would have included hunted duck, deer, and fish, and foraged vegetation like wild berries, nuts, and greens, but rather, we have thousands of choices—just not all of them are healthy ones. And lastly, the food itself has changed. Most of it isn't even actual food anymore.

What do I mean, it isn't food? Well, it depends on how you define what a food is. The dictionary definition of a food is "any *nutritious substance* that people or animals eat or drink or that plants absorb in order to *maintain life and growth*." I added the emphasis, as these are the key words: *nutritious substance* and *maintaining life and growth*. That should be what all foods do, by definition, right?

Let's look at this more closely. Our modern food supply is predominantly highly processed "food." It is combinations of ingredients that include additives, colorants, and chemicals and flavorings that have been specially designed to ensure that the "food" will last on a shelf for an extended period of time without spoiling, and also taste really good so that people will want to buy more of it. And one of the best ways to make something taste good is to—you guessed it—add sugar. (Sugar is also a great way to mask the disgusting taste of all the chemicals used to make products last longer on the shelf without spoiling.)

Although we call these items "food" because you can consume them, I don't consider them to be in the same category as actual food. Take the example in the illustration. We all agree that carrots

INGREDIENTS LISTS:
CARROTS COMPARED TO POP-TARTS®

Baby Carrots

Strawberry Banana Pop-Tart® Bites

Nutrition Facts

Serving size	(113g)

Amount per serving

Calories 40

	% Daily Value*
Total Fat 0g	**0%**
Saturated Fat 0g	**0%**
Trans Fat 0g	
Cholesterol 0mg	**0%**
Sodium 88mg	**4%**
Total Carbohydrate 9g	**3%**
Dietary Fiber 3g	**9%**
Total Sugars 5g	
Added Sugars	**0%**
Protein 1g	**1%**
Vitamin D 0mcg	0%
Calcium 36mg	4%
Iron 1mg	6%
Potassium 269mg	10%

*The % Daily Value (DV) tells you how much a nutrient in a serving of food contributes to a daily diet. 2,000 calories a day is used for general nutrition advice.

Ingredients: Baby Carrots

Nutrition Facts

Serving size	(40g)

Amount per serving

Calories 150

	% Daily Value*
Total Fat 4g	**5%**
Saturated Fat 2g	**10%**
Trans Fat 0g	
Cholesterol 0mg	**0%**
Sodium 160mg	**7%**
Total Carbohydrate 29g	**11%**
Dietary Fiber <1g	**2%**
Total Sugars 15g	
Added Sugars 15g	**30%**
Protein 1g	
Vitamin D 0mcg	0%
Calcium 0mg	0%
Iron 0.6mg	2%
Potassium 20mg	0%

*The % Daily Value (DV) tells you how much a nutrient in a serving of food contributes to a daily diet. 2,000 calories a day is used for general nutrition advice.

Ingredients: Enriched flour (wheat flour, niacin, reduced iron, vitamin B1 [thiamin mononitrate], vitamin B2 [riboflavin], folic acid), high fructose corn syrup, sugar, palm oil, glycerin. Contains 2% or less of strawberry puree concentrate, banana puree, modified tapioca starch, modified corn starch, salt, wheat flour, leavening (baking soda, sodium aluminum phosphate), cellulose, cornstarch, cellulose gel, natural and artificial flavors, cellulose gum, citric acid, sodium stearoyl lactylate, yellow 5 lake, soy lecithin, gelatin, wheat starch, DATEM, wheat gluten, red 40 lake, carrageenan, guar gum, red 40.

are a food. You can plant them in your yard. They contain nutrients that support our health. And when you look at the ingredients list, it is simple: carrots. It checks all of our dictionary-definition boxes for being a food: nutritious substance and maintains life and growth. But look at the Pop-Tarts®. First, there is no Pop-Tarts® tree where these are harvested. These are man-made creations and contain gelatin to give them a "goo" that melts a certain way in your mouth, and Red 40 Lake and Yellow 5 Lake, which are additives that make the goo a fun, pretty color. They also contain diacetyl tartaric acid ester of mono- and diglycerides to make sure the ingredients bind, as well as citric acid and cellulose gum to ensure they can stay on the shelf for a year or more. There is no nutritional need for us to consume wax, soy lecithin, or guar gum. Natural and artificial flavors don't support or maintain our life and growth; if anything, I would argue that they curtail it.

The Cost of Sugar Addiction

For some people, sugar addiction is a result of necessity. For many people these processed foods are the only reliable food option available. More Americans are living in what are known as food deserts, or poorer neighborhoods with limited access to fresh and healthy food. Low income and low access to food are the two features used to assess whether a region should be considered as a food desert.

It is also known that there's a correlation between poverty and obesity, and this is seen not only in the US, but globally. One study found that countries with poverty rates greater than 35 percent have obesity rates 145 percent higher than wealthy countries. Many families, due to financial reasons or lack of access, or both, are reliant on the corner convenience store as their primary place for purchasing food. And if you owned a small corner convenience store, would you stock it with products that will last a few months on the shelves, or with produce that only few people may want to buy, and that will rot in a few days? The profit margins point toward the shelf-stable items as being the safer bet. Overall, Americans have become reliant on fast and easy foods, sometimes as their only option.

Our mindset around sugar has also changed dramatically over the years. It used to be the case that a sweet treat was something you had on a special occasion, or once in a while. Now, we treat ourselves all day long. From morning until night, we are constantly scratching our sugar itch. We start our days with sugar-laden coffee drinks and cereals. At lunch, our healthy salad is drowned with salad dressing that we don't even realize contains sugar. Sports drinks or energy drinks with added sugar are followed by a dinner of pizza where there is sugar in the dough *and* the sauce. Dessert is every night. Parents, teachers, and pediatricians give kids candy for simply behaving, and worse, to make them feel better after a boo-boo. Sweets have become an expectation. Sugar is the new norm.

And we have the data to back all of this up. Americans are consuming more sugar than ever. Back in the 1750s, the average American consumed about 1 teaspoon of sugar per day. Compare that to today—we consume, per person, an average of 22 teaspoons per day!

Sugar Babies

While our food environment has changed, our brains have not. We have the same old brains of our starving hunters and gatherers who walked for hours to find one wild strawberry. But now, it is like we are living in a real-world version of the game Candy Land®. Sugar is everywhere we look, and ripe for the picking.

Our brains are like a kid in the candy store, with no one keeping shop. Our instincts to desire sugar lie in very primitive parts of our brain. This is the same place where other instinctual urges lie, like to mate or care for our young. The more evolved parts of the brain belong to the outer area (called the cortex), and this part of the brain helps to put the brakes on those primitive urges, so that we do them at the right time and in the right place. Our rational brain is what permits selection with our sexual partners, and also allows us to be able to leave our children with the babysitter.

When it comes to sugar, many of us have a hard time letting that rational part of the brain do its job. No matter what we say or do, it seems that our rational self is being overruled, and the primitive urges to eat sugar win. Why? And most importantly, how can we break free?

The reason many of us struggle with controlling our sugar intake is because it is addictive. Just like drugs or alcohol. I will be covering this more throughout the book, especially in chapter 3. One of the things that makes sugar more pervasive of an addiction than drugs or alcohol is that we were *born* craving it. Just like "crack babies"

OUR EVOLVING BRAIN

Our brains are complex, but we can visualize them based on how they have evolved. The inner portion is our "primitive brain" while the grayed portion can be considered our "rational brain."

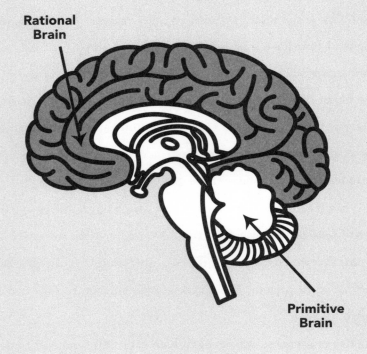

Rational Brain

Primitive Brain

are born physically dependent on crack cocaine because their moms used it during pregnancy. We all emerge into this world as little "sugar babies," with a biological desire to seek out sweets for safety and nourishment. Layer that onto our modern, sugar-soaked food supply and laissez-faire attitudes about food that promote eating sweets everywhere we go, and it's no wonder that so many people are addicted to sugar.

How can we break free? The answer to that question lies within the rest of this book. I am going to break down the science behind why and how people get addicted to sugar, so we can understand how to reverse it. I will also show you how you can use the power of psychology and learning to undo bad habits that we have developed as a society. But before we get to working on that, I want to talk a bit about *why* we need to get our sugar addiction under control before it's too late.

Diet Culture Dominance

By the time you get to the end of this chapter, you will see all of the ways in which sugar has invariably inflicted its damage on us. But before we get into that, we should address the primary way in which it enters our lives: through diet culture.

Diet culture has continually fueled us as a society to be in constant states of hunger or overconsuming. This isn't new—it dates back to the early part of the 1900s, when the general public became introduced to calories and counting them as a way of controlling your waistline. Then, in the 1920s, smoking cigarettes was popularized as the best way to control your weight, followed by calorie counting in the 1950s, and the emergence of WeightWatchers® in the 1960s.

It was also diet culture that, in the 1970s, told us that fat will make you "fat" and give you heart disease. Diet culture ate up this information, because it was science-backed and allowed companies and the media to market products as "good" or "bad" foods. Products high in fat on the nutrition label were no longer selling at the rates they had before, leading to further diet culture infiltration. But during this time, no one was concerned about how many carbohydrates they were consuming due to the message that the "bad" food at the time was fats. As I mentioned in the introduction, diet culture began to push carbohydrate-heavy lifestyles, for "heart health." What wasn't generally known at that time was that sugar, a carbohydrate, contributes just as much to heart disease development as saturated fats do.

Diet culture has a lot of control over our behaviors. The confusion sets in when every few years (or more often) there seems to be a new set of messages and advice to follow: eat low fat, eat high protein, fast in the mornings, fast at night, eat only plants, eat only meat, and on and on. For decades, brands and the media have pushed specific diets on the public, yet the obesity epidemic is still increasing.

Why? The toxic appeal of "losing ten pounds in a week" has made Americans believe in a quick fix. Cleanses, yo-yo dieting, or cutting out entire food groups completely are often portrayed as the magical cure for your weight loss woes. But diet studies have shown that this isn't accurate—especially when it comes to cutting out entire food groups (like carbohydrates). The bottom line is that there is no magic bullet or quick fix, and the diet culture narrative portrayed in our society is doing much more harm than good.

Sugar Is a Silent Killer

What does that mean? It means that sugar is harming you, and it isn't always obvious. This is why parents don't often see the harm in letting their kids overeat sweets. This is also why many people who struggle with bingeing on sugar might be able to deny that their bingeing is a problem. If your doctor says that you're healthy, your bloodwork is normal, etc., then you are healthy, right? You might be healthy, for now. The negative consequences of overeating sugar don't appear overnight. They can take decades to emerge in the form of heart disease, cognitive impairments, obesity, or cancer. In fact, a recent study found that consumption of added sugar has been linked to forty-five different negative health outcomes! Often by the time these conditions manifest, the damage has already been done.

Let's Weigh In on Weight

Just because someone is overeating (meaning, eating more calories than they intend to, or more calories than they can burn off) doesn't mean that they are destined to become overweight or obese. There are many factors that can contribute to obesity and becoming overweight—overeating is just one of them. Metabolism, age, genetics, how much you exercise, and sometimes just darn luck also play a role.

We tend to focus on the health dangers that can come from being overweight or obese (more on this in a few pages), but does that mean that overeating is okay if you don't gain weight from it? No way! Overeating has psychological and emotional effects that can be just as debilitating. I will cover some of these later in this chapter.

Because we are designed to like to eat sugar, and because sugar is everywhere, *and*, as I'll explain in more detail in chapter 3, sugar is addictive, we overeat it. Some of us know we overeat it, while others overeat and are less aware or unaware that we're doing it, because we don't have any overt warnings (like being overweight or obese, or having any health complications as a result, at least not yet). Overeating is common, but it is also complicated. It is hard to understand because it can be triggered by so many different things. Stress is a common source of overeating, and so is anxiety. In fact, self-medication with food has become a common way in which people cope with the struggles of daily life. In a study looking at nutritional and behavioral factors that induce eating of "comfort foods" in response to stress, women who used such "comfort foods" reported a reduction in their perceived stress compared to those who do not engage in eating foods in this way. Many Americans fall into a cycle of consuming hyperpalatable "comfort" food to self-medicate, often followed by overconsumption of all foods. No one is going to self-medicate their stress with a salad. Specific foods, "comfort foods"—like potato chips, ice cream, cookies, candy, pizza, and pasta—are what people reach for when they are seeking a way to self-soothe with food. While there are many reasons (in addition to self-medication) why people overeat, there is one common denominator that we tend to see when it comes to the *types* of foods people overeat: they usually contain added sugar.

Weight Is Not Synonymous with Health

Human beings come in all shapes and sizes and should be loved and accepted regardless of how they look. It's great that we are seeing more inclusivity of larger bodies in advertising. Since most people in the United States *are* overweight or obese, the majority of people buying clothes are larger people. Therefore, it makes sense that there should be larger-bodied mannequins to model clothes. Some argue that obese mannequins further normalize an unhealthy body weight and create a new "ideal." I don't agree with this position at all. Stores just want to sell clothes and make money, so it makes great business sense to have their models represent their population of shoppers. It isn't the Gap® or Athleta®'s job to teach us about our health ideals. The mannequins are modeling the clothes, not our health.

The fact is that weight is not synonymous with health. Not in the least.

Some of the unhealthiest people I have met and worked with have been what would be considered a "healthy weight." Yet they were totally addicted to sugar, and were bingeing on it regularly. They weren't happy. They felt out of control. They wanted to change their behavior but felt stuck. And since they didn't have their doctor telling them they needed to lose weight or felt that they were normal weight, this dug them deeper and deeper into their sugar pit.

People with obesity are victims of our toxic diet culture and food environment that has shifted us away from eating actual food and made us reliant on processed food, which in turn has led many to become addicted to sugar, and *that* is what's contributing to the rise in obesity. I'll get into the details on how (and why) this has happened in later chapters, but for now just note that I'm not shaming or blaming people for being overweight or obese. To me, that would be the equivalent of shaming or blaming someone for having seasonal allergies. Hey, they have to breathe, and they can't help it that there are trees and flowers in their area that mess with their respiratory system. Just like humans must eat food, and we can't help it if our food supply is dominated by foods that, by design, will make us obese. Plus, unlike other addictive things, like drugs and alcohol, we *need* food to survive, so going without it is not an option.

I am, however, against the health problems and chronic conditions that are directly linked to obesity. Obesity is a chronic illness that is diagnosed typically by using body mass index (BMI) and other inflammatory markers including blood glucose, triglycerides, and waist-to-hip circumference. Obesity is categorized as a chronic condition due to the plethora of other conditions that accompany or follow an obesity diagnosis. Cancers, cardiovascular disease, diabetes, sleep apnea, and muscle wasting are all comorbidities of obesity. Metabolic disorder is another one of the many complications that come with obesity. This syndrome is characterized by certain clinical manifestations, including increased blood pressure, blood sugar, excess body fat around the waist (central adiposity), and abnormal cholesterol and triglyceride levels. What makes this so crucial to clinical care is the outcomes. Metabolic syndrome leads to further metabolic damage, like insulin resistance, which is the body's inabilty to use insulin properly. This then leads to trouble in all areas of life. The prevalence in the United States of metabolic syndrome is 30 percent and growing. The main issue in the United States still stands with the fact that most people and doctors are doing little, if anything at all, about reducing or preventing this from happening in the first place. And restaurants, the diet industry, and social media are only making the obesity epidemic worse.

Most people know that obesity and being overweight pose huge health risks, but rates continue to rise. We know what obesity is and what it can do, we accept it, and as a society we have normalized it. Although over 39 percent of the US population was obese in 2016, there has been little change in our healthcare system to address this. Fueled by stressors of the pandemic, obesity rates stood at 42.4 percent of all Americans in 2020. We are in crisis mode. So why isn't anyone doing anything about it?

WHAT'S WRONG WITH BMI?

The use of BMI to diagnose someone as being overweight or obese has its limits, and it isn't always accurate. First, it is just a measure of weight and height, and it doesn't account for muscle mass versus fat accrual. Professional athletes, like football players, can be considered overweight or obese according to their BMI, even though they are likely very low in body fat. Similarly, many people who work out regularly and have larger muscles can be mislabeled as being overweight or obese for this reason. That is why it is important to consider BMI within the context of other markers for health—including blood markers (like cholesterol, insulin, or glucose levels). BMI is just one measure of health—not the only one.

Why Overeating Is Beating Us

Several things are happening in concert that are allowing obesity to win. First, the average American is overweight or obese. When you look around you and many other people are this way, it seems normal. If something is the norm, it can't be bad for us, right? Second, people are burnt out by diet culture. For decades they have been told by the media, celebrities, and diet gurus to follow one diet or another, and none of them really work. Or if they do work, the weight comes back soon after you go off the diet. Lastly, sugar is a drug. We use it and abuse it just like some people use and abuse other drugs, like alcohol or heroin. Bad day at work? Get a sugary coffee drink. Stressed about your in-laws coming to visit? Eat a piece of cake. Sugar-rich foods are a socially acceptable and legal way of making ourselves feel good. But like other addictive substances, that is just half of the reason why we use them. Addiction lures us in by making us feel good at first, but over time, as the addiction takes hold of us, we need to use the substance just to feel normal.

Sugar's Role in Chronic Disease

Over the years government organizations have warned of the dangers of a diet high in sugar and have urged people to cut back to prevent chronic diseases. Unfortunately, far too many people have ignored this guidance; as a result, many chronic diseases have become more prevalent. Epidemiological studies suggest that excess sugar is associated with chronic diseases, including type 2 diabetes (T2DM), cardiovascular disease (CVD), and cancer, and often the medical advice for each of these illnesses highlights the importance of reducing added sugars. Let's take a closer look at some of the medical conditions that have been linked to sugar intake, so we can understand how a simple shift in the way we eat can have a significant impact on our health in many different ways.

IS SUGAR THE NEW TOBACCO?

Food companies are often considered "the bad guys," and in many cases rightly so, often sacrificing our health for their profit margins. If sugar is added to their products, they taste better (more on this in chapter 2). A bonus for them is that consumers can easily become addicted, much like the tobacco industry. Most tobacco products are sold legally, but people make the decision to buy them. The argument is that everyone (at least nowadays) knows tobacco is bad for you and addictive, so if you go ahead and buy cigarettes and get hooked on them, that's on you.

Even the tobacco industry admits that their products are addictive (see the warning labels and public health campaigns they sponsor). But food companies don't admit potential negative health effects or slap a warning label on their products.

The closest to a warning about sugar was in 2015 when the FDA set a rule that companies need to disclose the amount of added sugar in their products on the Nutrition Facts label. But the clever food companies figured their way out of that by changing their formulations to include sweeteners that are still bad for you and addictive, though aren't considered "added sugars" by the FDA. For a list of these and what we know from the science about what they can do to your brain and body, see chapter 2.

Tobacco isn't hidden in my yogurt, but sugar is. It isn't in my breakfast cereal, but sugar is. Tobacco isn't in drinks with cute Disney® characters on the labels, but sugar is. See my point?

Added sugar is also found in things that are purposely placed at eye level in stores. This isn't a joke—grocery store space is like luxury real estate shopping. Think of the endcaps and main eye-level shelves being the equivalent of oceanfront property. Companies pay top dollar to have their products in those spots. The less sexy, poorer brands (that are often the healthier options) are way up top or way on the bottom, where you can barely reach them or are too lazy to bend down. Companies know that the average person hitting the grocery store is typically a woman with a kid or two in tow, who probably wants to get in and out of there as fast as possible without any drama. Or it's someone in a rush, who just wants to grab the food without having to hunt around for the healthiest options. Big brands with the most money place the foods they want to push right in front of us (or our kids). They are taking advantage of us.

Type 2 Diabetes Mellitus

The realization that excess sugar and T2DM are correlated dates all the way back to 1907. Despite this observation from over a hundred years ago, government agencies are still begging people to reduce their sugar intake to prevent T2DM while the food industry keeps formulating highly processed sugary foods that add to that risk. Briefly, T2DM is a chronic condition where your body cannot properly metabolize the sugar you consume. This leads to high blood sugar levels, also known as hyperglycemia. If hyperglycemia isn't managed, it can lead to a host of complications, including nerve damage, kidney failure, and loss of eyesight. While we know that too much sugar is *associated* with T2DM, it can't be blamed as the sole cause, as not everyone who eats a lot of sugar gets this disease. Plus, it is still debated how much sugar alone is to blame for the increasing rates of T2DM, and whether obesity resulting from a poor diet is actually more at fault. But we do know that sugar carries its own risk factor for developing T2DM. For every serving of sugar-sweetened beverage per day, the risk of developing T2DM increases by 27 percent.

Ultra-processed foods share in the responsibility for developing T2DM as well. Much of the population gets a large portion of their calories from ultra-processed foods, and a majority of people's sugar intake comes from these products. This is alarming because for every 10 percent incremental increase of ultra-processed food intake, there's a 25 percent higher risk of developing T2DM. In addition to sugar-sweetened beverages and ultra-processed foods contributing to T2DM incidents, refined carbohydrates can be harmful too. Our body digests and processes refined carbs into sugar quickly—foods like white bread, refined grains, and pastas. These foods are classified as high glycemic index (GI) foods, and reducing them has been shown to help with overall glucose control in people who have a diagnosis of T2DM. When you review much of the data out there, the message is pretty straightforward: avoiding sugar can help lessen your risk of getting T2DM, and if you already have it, avoiding it will help keep your blood glucose levels under control.

Cardiovascular Disease

CVD is the umbrella term for several heart diseases, including coronary artery disease (CAD), heart failure, hypertension (high blood pressure), stroke, and peripheral artery disease (PAD). These conditions are often caused by a buildup of plaque, which blocks blood vessels in the body; all that can be partially blamed on excess sugar in the diet. CVD is so common, chances are you or a loved one are affected by this disease. In fact, it is the most common cause of death in the US, and just like many other chronic ailments, it can also be tied back to too much sugar. Although the risk of CVD is influenced by other factors such as diet (red and particularly processed meat consumption has been linked to greater risk of CVD), genetics, race, and gender, and while you can't change your biology, you can change what you eat and drink. But even if you're at higher risk of CVD because of your family history or your gender (men are at greater risk than women), just know that sugar's influence on CVD does not discriminate: studies show that sugar intake increases the risk of CVD across all age groups, most races/ethnicities, and sex, and that increase is pretty high. Each serving per day incrementally ups your risk of CVD by 9 to 11 percent! If you think that's bad, two or more servings per day increases your risk of dying from CVD by over 30 percent.

The first line of prevention of CVD is a healthful diet, and as you may have guessed, the medical advice recommended for CVD is to limit "ultra-processed carbohydrates and sugar-sweetened beverages." Historically, when it came to heart health, people were told to stay away from *trans* fats and cholesterol, but now we know sugar isn't good for our heart either. Besides causing your liver to create fat, increasing inflammation and uric acid, and contributing to dysregulated blood sugar levels (all of which can contribute to developing CVD), too much sugar also causes the fat cells around the membrane of your heart to build up (aka pericardial adipose tissue), further heightening the risk of CVD. Since sugar attacks the heart through different mechanisms, limiting your intake of it, in all its processed and sneaky forms, is one important way to keep your heart healthy.

Cancer

About 40 percent of cancers diagnosed in the United States are associated with obesity. Although the association is not seen across all types of cancer, as of now there are thirteen cancers that can be directly associated with being overweight and obesity. It is true that cancer cells *love* sugar. Cancer cells grow and divide at a much faster pace than other cells in our body, which explains why they take in so much sugar for fuel. But this doesn't necessarily mean that the sugar from our foods "feeds" the cancer cells. While there's still plenty of research that needs to be conducted to understand the complex relationship between dietary factors and tumor growth, there's lots of research already out there supporting a strong association between sugar and cancer. One reason for this relationship may be due to the pro-inflammatory nature of sugar. Inflammation can damage the DNA in our cells, which leads to shoddy replication and gene mutations, leading to cancer. Another is that sugar stimulates the secretion of insulin and insulin-like growth factors, both of which can promote tumor growth and progression. This may partially explain why one large study analyzing dietary information from over 100,000 participants found those with the highest total sugar intake had the highest risk of cancer.

The risk associated with sugar-sweetened beverage consumption and cancer is a finding worth throwing your sugar-sweetened drink of choice right down the drain. In those with central adiposity (aka overweight in the midsection), higher sugary beverage intake is associated with almost a 60 percent higher risk of obesity-related cancers. Furthermore, sugar-sweetened beverages have been positively associated with death from *all* cancers, especially breast cancer. For men, across all races, who consume the highest amount of sugar from beverages, their risk of prostate cancer jumps to 21 percent.

Alzheimer's Disease and Poorer Cognitive Function

If reading about all the ways that sugar can harm your health and contribute to diseases isn't enough to convince you to ditch it, there's more. Sugar intake can affect your *brain* health.

The blood-brain barrier is a filter that surrounds the brain to protect it from toxins and other harmful compounds in the bloodstream, while also providing the brain with important nutrients it needs to function, including glucose (a type of sugar that our cells use for fuel). The brain utilizes about 20 percent of the body's total glucose requirement. Glucose can enter the brain through different transport proteins. Under normal circumstances, the brain gets the glucose it needs to carry out functions including energy production, synthesis of neurotransmitters, and fighting off oxidative stress (which, if not combated, can lead to damage in our tissues, DNA, and proteins). However, during periods of hyperglycemia or dysfunctional glucose metabolism, excess amounts of glucose can pass through the blood-brain barrier, which can be toxic to the brain. To put it scientifically, too much sugar impairs your cognitive functioning. To put it bluntly, too much sugar makes you dumb.

Unfortunately, the damage that sugar can inflict on the cognitive function can begin even before birth. One study utilizing food intake questionnaires found children born to mothers who ate a high-sugar diet and drank sugar-sweetened beverages while pregnant had poorer cognition and nonverbal abilities to solve problems. Maternal sugar intake during breastfeeding can also negatively impact the developing brain of her baby. A negative association has been found in mothers who consumed high amounts of sugar-sweetened beverages and juice at the first postnatal month and neurodevelopment outcomes in the babies even two years later.

It gets worse. Larger intakes of unhealthy foods high in added sugars are associated with smaller hippocampal volume as well as impaired memory and learning. The hippocampus is one of the brain regions that is essential for proper learning and memory—and studies suggest that sugar can *shrink* it. In addition, childhood sugar-sweetened beverage consumption is negatively associated with verbal intelligence at mid-childhood.

Research has shown that adults with high sugar intake score significantly lower on cognitive tests compared to those who eat less sugar. Although most of the sugar from this particular study came from sugar-sweetened beverages, processed foods and desserts are also to blame. However, sugar-sweetened beverages seem to be the riskiest to consume, as they were responsible for an almost four times higher risk of cognitive impairment compared with sugar from other sources. Furthermore, adults who consume more than 11 teaspoons of sugar per day are also more likely to score lower on immediate and delayed memory tests, as well as verbal memory, which allows us

SWEETNESS OF YOUTH

Looking back, did you overdo the sugar as a kid? If so, don't fret. Limiting sugar during early life and childhood may be a beneficial strategy in optimizing brain function and preserving brain volume. Unfortunately, you can't climb into the time machine. Don't worry if when reflecting on your childhood diet you realize you consumed a lot more sugar than you should have. The brain is malleable, and making healthful changes later in life will still be beneficial for brain health.

to hear, process, store, and recall information. Although 11 teaspoons of sugar may sound like a lot, to put it into perspective, it's actually less than the amount of sugar in a 20-oz bottle of Coke®.

Recent studies have also suggested a link between excessive sugar intake and the development of dementia. In fact, due to this link, some have even begun to consider whether Alzheimer's disease should be called "type 3 diabetes." Persistent hyperglycemia, found in individuals who have T2DM and prediabetes, has been shown to be associated with developing dementia and cognitive impairment. While the exact causes of neurodegeneration that occurs in people with diabetes remain to be seen, periods of hyperglycemia have been shown to cause an inflammatory response within the brain. Just like other cells in the body, there are insulin receptors within the limbic system of the brain. Although the brain is not dependent on insulin to maintain glucose levels, insulin plays a vital role in regulating cognitive functions including attention, memory, and learning. Therefore, high sugar levels with concurrent insulin resistance may partially explain why dysfunction of insulin signaling has been associated with Alzheimer's disease. Furthermore, worse memory and attention performance, as well as a decrease in brain gray matter, are associated with T2DM. In fact, those with a longer duration of T2DM are more likely to have dementia and mild cognitive impairment. People with chronic hyperglycemia in T2DM have a higher risk of getting Alzheimer's disease, which may be partially due to high glucose levels contributing to neuroinflammation and brain injury.

If you don't have diabetes, don't think you're off the hook from developing cognitive impairment—high blood sugar in the absence of a diagnosis of diabetes is also problematic. In these cases, hyperglycemia alone has been associated with poorer cognitive function and atrophy of the hippocampus, further supporting the detrimental impact a high-sugar diet has on the brain as a whole. Like soda intake being associated with increased risk of depression (see next section), higher sweet beverage intake, including juice, is associated with preclinical signs of Alzheimer's disease. Just two sugary drinks per day are equivalent to two years of brain aging when compared to abstaining from these drinks completely. One drink per day, including fruit juice, is also associated with less total brain volume, hippocampal volume, and poorer performance on episodic memory tests.

In summary, regardless of age, overconsumption of sugar potentially contributes to an array of deleterious effects in the brain. While many of the mechanisms are still being uncovered, avoiding hidden sugars in food is a way to help promote overall brain health and function.

Mental Health

We often use sugar to attempt to self-medicate our mental health issues, like mild-moderate depression and anxiety, but in reality, added sugar is often *promoting* mental unwellness. Although the underlying causes of many mental health conditions are out of our control, like genetics and our biochemical makeup, there *are* things in our control that increase or decrease our risk. For example, drugs and alcohol are modifiable risk factors that are directly correlated with many mental health conditions like depression, anxiety, and ADHD. Drugs of abuse can cause changes in the brain that directly contribute to a person developing a mental health condition. So it shouldn't be much of a surprise to learn that just like drugs and alcohol, too much sugar may also place you at a higher risk since it affects your brain in a similar fashion. Let's look at the science behind how nutrition, and sugar in particular, can impact some of the common mental health conditions that arise.

Depression. Clinical depression can occur at any age and is one of the most common mental health conditions in the US. Just like other mental health disorders, there are many underlying factors that can increase one's risk of developing depression, and sugar is no exception. In fact, drinking two cups of soda per day—that's just *one* small-size soda at a fast-food restaurant—may increase your risk for depression by 5 percent. If you think that's bad, three cans per day might increase your risk by 25 percent. Other studies have shown that just one sugar-sweetened beverage per day is associated with a higher prevalence of major depressive disorder.

Although soda is often the main source of sugar in most people's diets, poor-quality carbohydrates from processed foods can also impact mood and depression. Researchers set out to see the association between the glycemic load of a diet with mood disturbances and risk of depression. Assessing glycemic load in studies allows researchers to measure the quality and quantity of a carbohydrate. High glycemic load diets contain more refined grains and added sugars and resemble more of a Western style diet, while low glycemic load diets have more carbs coming from healthier sources, like whole grains. After assigning people either a high or low glycemic load diet, researchers found that people who consumed the high glycemic load diet scored 40 percent higher on depression symptom assessments compared to those who were assigned to the low glycemic load diet. Another study followed people for ten years and found that those who ate the most added sugars from processed carbohydrates and drinks had the highest risk of depression. While based on these studies we can't say that sugar is *causing* depression, it certainly is associated with putting people at higher risk.

Anxiety. Although it is normal to worry or be fearful some of the time, when living with an anxiety disorder, the fear and anxiety don't ever go away. The excessive dread and irrational fear can grow and, in some cases, can cause severe impairments. Anxiety is one of the most prevalent mental health conditions in the US. Approximately 31 percent of adults report they have experienced an anxiety disorder at some point in their lifetime.

Just like other mental health conditions, you probably guessed that sugar plays a role in anxiety as well. Studies have found that individuals with high levels of anxiety eat significantly more sugar compared to those with low levels of anxiety. In addition, a study found that those who consumed a higher-than-average amount of ultra-processed food (think soda, cakes, cereals—all foods with lots of added sugars) have a higher prevalence of anxiety compared to people who consumed more minimally processed foods. This is similar to other findings showing that those who consumed a dietary pattern containing more added sugars were more likely to have higher levels of anxiety, compared to those who consumed diets with minimal added sugars.

There are a few different mechanisms through which sugar may exacerbate anxiety. For one, sugar can cause erratic fluctuations in blood glucose levels, and poor glycemic control is associated with higher levels of anxiety. In addition, sugar can have an impact on our gut flora (aka our microbiome), promoting low-grade inflammation. This, in turn, negatively impacts our brain health. Briefly (because this can be a chapter on its own), the gut and brain communicate with each other through what is known as the gut-brain axis. Basically, too much added sugar alters the gut microbes, which compromises the communication to the brain and increases inflammation, in turn impacting mental health and anxiety levels. Lastly, some people use sugar to manage their anxiety—self-medicating with sugar can be a way for people to temporarily feel better, but in the long run it just makes their anxiety worse. Taken together, it makes sense why a high-sugar diet is often associated with anxiety. Although dietary changes are not currently one of the established treatment modalities for anxiety, mostly due to lack of research or intervention studies in this area, limiting sugar, or completely removing it, is likely to be impactful, and many psychiatrists recommend cutting back on sugar if you are having trouble with anxiety.

Attention-Deficit/Hyperactivity Disorder. Similar to how sugar intake and obesity rates have soared over the last twenty years, the rates of attention-deficit/hyperactivity disorder (ADD/ADHD) have also risen precipitously during this same time frame. Although the causes of ADHD are controversial and multifactorial, one of them may be related to neuroinflammation. So, if neuroinflammation could be contributing to ADHD, you can see why sugar may be contributing to this increase, or at least making it worse. Sugar can lead to an inflammatory response not only in the gut, as discussed earlier in this chapter, but also in other parts of the body and brain.

Often, we think of ADHD as a childhood disorder, but many of the symptoms and impairments of this disorder often continue into adulthood. And while much of the research examining the relationship between diet and ADHD is done in children, when you stop and think about it, that research most likely applies to adults since we probably had lots of sugar as kids, too! Some studies show that there is a relationship between dietary patterns typically loaded with refined carbohydrates and sugar and a diagnosis of ADHD. But the findings are conflicting. While some studies have shown a relationship between sugar intake and ADHD, others have not. However, a clinical study suggests that the sugar your mom consumed while pregnant has a lasting impact on you, too: intrauterine exposure to just one or more cups of sweet beverages per day is associated with ADHD symptoms in offspring. That's a pretty good reason to avoid soda during pregnancy! And even though we can't say for sure that sugar directly causes ADHD, one thing we can probably agree on is that sugar makes people hyper and may make the symptoms worse.

Premature Death

We all want to live as long as possible. And there is a huge market for longevity—everywhere you turn there seems to be a new product that claims to make you look or feel younger and more vibrant. While looking and feeling younger is always a plus, how to live longer is a topic of interest for many researchers. Up until recently it was a long-held belief that genetics was the main determinant of one's life span. However, this is no longer the case, and now we know that only about 7 percent of our life span can be attributed to our genetic makeup. Since only a small fraction of our life expectancy is completely out of our hands, more weight is given to the factors that are within our control. If you want to add almost ten years to your life, you're in luck. According to research out of Harvard, there are five lifestyle-related factors that can help you get there: following a healthy dietary pattern, not smoking, drinking alcohol in moderation, making physical activity part of your routine, and maintaining your weight. People who consistently follow these factors are more likely to live longer. Unfortunately, only about 8 percent of the entire US population adheres to this "low-risk" lifestyle. Let's take a more detailed look at the first factor: following a healthy dietary pattern.

A healthy diet isn't just about what we eat—what we drink matters, too. We know that drinking sugar-sweetened beverages increases your risk for different chronic diseases (see previous sections), but did you know that it also puts you at risk of dying earlier? One large analysis including over thirty-five studies found that every 250 ml increase in daily sugar-sweetened beverage intake increases your risk of mortality by 4 percent. To put that in perspective, that's not even a full can of soda. Another large study found that sugar-sweetened beverage intake, even after taking into account BMI, dietary, and lifestyle factors, increases your risk of dying.

If you're thinking that you can just swap in some artificially sweetened beverages to boost your life span, think again. Research shows that these types of beverages also contribute to reduced life expectancy. And it isn't just the beverages that we need to be mindful about. Ultra-processed foods are so bad for our longevity that more than four servings per day is associated with a 62 percent increased hazard for all causes of death. If you think that's bad, every additional serving tacks on another 18 percent hazard risk. There are other ingredients besides sugar in these products, so we can't only single out sugar when looking at the research results of these foods. However, we don't eat nutrients in isolation, and most of these foods contain some form of sugar.

Taken together, if someone eats ultra-processed foods and drinks sugar-sweetened beverages or juices, all that sugar can add up quickly, chiseling off years of life! A diet where more than 20 percent of the calories comes from sugar increases the risk of dying by 30 percent. Keep in mind, the majority of Americans already eat a diet that contains at least 13 percent sugar-derived calories. While we still haven't figured out all the secrets to extend life, we can confidently say that too much sugar shortens it.

▶●◀

I know this chapter makes me sound like a real downer with all of the gloom and doom about what your sugar intake has been doing to your health, but the good news is this can be within your control. It's not just about skipping the cupcakes, but also being smart and knowing where sugar lurks. Now is the time to start making changes so that you can avoid it moving forward and improve your health and happiness. Let's start off by taking a closer look at our foe, sugar, so you can better understand all the places it is lurking and sneaking into your diet.

CHAPTER 2

SUGAR IS HIDING IN PLAIN SIGHT

One factor that makes cutting back on sugar so difficult is that it isn't always obvious where it is lurking. Many foods that appear to be healthy are often loaded with sugar. In this chapter, we'll review the places where sugar is hiding, go over all the aliases and pseudonyms used by the food industry, and debunk some myths about the "healthier" sugars you probably see listed on ingredient labels (spoiler alert: they are still sugar and bad for you).

Burning Questions About the Sweet Stuff

Sugar is a sneaky little ingredient, and for nefarious reasons, it finds its way into products where we would least expect it. But before we get into all of that, let me first address a few of the most common questions I get about the sweet stuff. They may be the reason why you picked up this book in the first place!

What is a sugar? And why do we need it? It should be a simple answer, but it can get complicated.

A sugar is a carbohydrate. But this doesn't mean that *sugar* and *carbohydrate* are synonymous. Nor does it mean that if you are trying to reduce your added sugar intake you need to cut back on *all* carbohydrates, or even all foods containing sugars naturally (like fruit). Let me explain why.

All carbohydrates eventually are broken down in our bodies into, among other nutrients, glucose (a type of sugar). Glucose is the energy that is essential for life. It is the fuel for our cells and is used throughout our bodies. Some glucose is used immediately as energy. If it is not used immediately, our bodies store glucose in a different form, called glycogen. When we need extra energy, like when we rigorously exercise, our bodies can use the glycogen stockpiles and turn them into energy. It's a clever way in which our bodies have evolved so that we don't have to eat nonstop to have energy—we can store it up for future use.

Some argue that since carbohydrates break down in our bodies into sugars, they should be viewed in the same way as other sugars. I don't agree with that logic. Here is why: You could eat zero carbohydrates and your body would just *make* sugar as a fuel (thanks to your liver!). This occurs through a process called gluconeogenesis (translation: gluco = sugar, neo = new, genesis = make, or "make new sugar"). Our cells need glucose, a sugar that is a necessary body fuel, to survive. And if we aren't eating foods that contain carbohydrates that can easily be made into glucose, our bodies will just make it from non-carbohydrate sources such as protein, lactate from our muscles, and fatty acids.

Blood glucose levels must be maintained within a narrow range for good health. If blood sugar is too high, it results in tissue and organ damage. If it is too low, cellular respiration and energy production can suffer. Therefore, the ability of our bodies to "make new sugar" and regulate blood sugar levels is critical. The main advantage of this process is that it helps the body maintain steady blood sugar levels when foods containing carbohydrates or stored sugars (glycogen reserves) are unavailable. Without gluconeogenesis, you wouldn't live long, especially without food, as your body needs a constant and steady level of blood glucose to keep the brain and red blood cells going. This is also how people who eat a strict keto diet, which offers very few carbohydrates, are still alive.

So the bottom line is, no matter what you eat, like it or not, sugar is a by-product. And, for the reasons described above, that is a good thing. We need sugar in our bodies for them to work, and if we don't get it from our diet, our bodies will make it for us. Either way, we need sugar to live.

But here's the catch: we don't need *added* sugar to live. If anything, it's the added sugar that is slowly killing us. When I talk about reducing sugar, I'm talking about reducing intake of *added* sugar. There is a very big difference between the impact that added sugar has on our brain and behavior and what happens when someone consumes other carbohydrates. Also, as you will see in the next sections, many carbohydrate-containing foods that we consume are advantageous to our health and contain nutrients that we need to stay healthy, sans the added sugar.

Do I have to completely give up sugar, like, all of it? Cold turkey?! Nope! For most people, systematically identifying, replacing, and reducing sugar in your diet will help you to break your dependence on it.

So now you might be wondering, how can you still use something if you are addicted to it? Isn't it essential to completely quit something you're addicted to in order to recover? People aren't advised to do *less* drugs, like alcohol or cocaine—they must ditch them completely! This is true, to some extent. Yes, many people need to completely remove drugs or alcohol from their life to avoid the harm. However, with drugs or alcohol, it is easier in the sense that we can clearly identify them and avoid them. They aren't hidden in our foods, or constantly being pushed on us or marketed to us. Can you imagine what it would be like if you were trying to avoid using cocaine, but it was hidden in breakfast cereal, condiments, and other foods; everywhere you looked there were ads for it; and your friends were offering it to you constantly and questioning why you didn't want any?

The reality is that it's more complicated when it comes to sugar. We need food to survive, and many foods that are good for us—like fruits, some vegetables, and milks—naturally contain sugars that, in the amounts that they have, aren't bad for us. Plus, as you will learn throughout the rest of this chapter, sugar is hidden in so many places that you need to be a detective to find it all.

The all-or-nothing approach just sets you up for failure. No one, especially in our modern food environment, can successfully navigate our food landscape and escape *all* added sugar. As you will learn in this chapter, sugar is pervasive and is hidden by different names and for different reasons in our food supply. Expecting to completely avoid it just isn't reasonable or realistic. And we shouldn't beat ourselves up about eating it when we didn't intend to with all of this in the background.

What about quitting cold turkey? Over my years doing research in this area and talking with many people who have gone through an addiction to sugar, I have learned that the cold-turkey approach doesn't always work. Not to say that it *can't* work, but for most people it often brings with it a sense of failure and shame when people can't stick with it. Also, my psychology and neuroscience training has taught me that learning theory tells us that the cold-turkey approach isn't the best strategy in most cases for long-term change. If you want to reform your habits, it's best to do it incrementally. Don't worry, I'll show you how to do this as we move through the book.

What about other carbs? Aren't those sugars, too? Do I have to reduce my intake of all carbohydrates in order to break my addiction? Carbohydrates, in general, have gotten a bad rap. Despite what others may tell you, carbohydrates in general are *not* bad for you. Some incredibly healthy things—like apples, berries, and oats—contain carbohydrates. When you eat these types of carbs, your body knows what to do. It isn't the carbohydrates, per se, that are bad for you, it's the added sugar.

But then there's the question about those *other* carbs, like the breads and the pastas, that some people struggle to control their intake of. You might feel like you should restrict those as well, and you may have tried that already in the past and found it to be too difficult.

Some people end up so dependent on added sugars that even non-sweet sugars, like those we would find in other carbohydrate-rich foods, such as breads and pastas, can trigger them to overeat. I'll get into why this happens in the first place in the next sections, but it has to do with how carbohydrates are broken down by our bodies into "sugars" that we use as energy. Even though all carbohydrates end up as sugars in our bloodstream once they are broken down by our bodies, the process, and the outcome of how we feel as a result, differs depending on the type of sugar we are eating.

However, my experience is that most people are able to get a handle on their carbohydrate intake once they drastically cut back on the added sweet sugars. So in this book I don't adopt a no-carb policy for breaking your sugar addiction, as I believe that some carbohydrate-containing foods (like fruits, for example) can actually *help* wean you off of the added sugar. I don't advise cutting out, or even way back on, carbs like breads and pasta (unless you feel like you can't moderate them without a problem). As I mentioned above, first try cutting back on the added sugars and see how your body and brain react to that. You may find that you're craving these types of carbs much less after you give up the sweet stuff!

Also, you will see that some of the recipes I have created for you (see pp. 214–268) contain carbohydrates (but with some variations in case you're trying to reduce those, too, or just want to try something different). In chapter 5, I'll introduce some Craving Crushing foods that can help you to manage your sugar cravings—and many of them contain some carbohydrates.

What should I do if I crave it all: the sweet stuff, the bread, and the pastas? Some people have a sweet tooth, while others are more drawn toward breads, pastas, crackers, etc., which are high in carbohydrates, but not always sweet. Others are in the middle and find that both types of carbs (sweet and non-sweet) set them down the path of bingeing and craving. Which one are you? Take the quiz to find out. Knowing which types of foods are problematic for you is helpful in starting to change your habits.

Although cravings for carbohydrates come in the form of a sweet tooth for many people, it is not uncommon to crave non-sweet carbohydrate options, like bread or pasta. Why is this? Despite the type

WHAT TYPE OF CARBS DO YOU CRAVE?

FOR EACH PAIR. CIRCLE THE FOOD THAT YOU PREFER.

Sweet Carbs		Non-sweet Carbs
chocolate cake		pasta
ice cream		bread
frosted doughnut		cheese crackers
pudding		soft pretzels
milkshake	**OR**	potato chips
muffins		bagels
cookies		croissants
brownies		tortilla chips
apple pie		pizza
chocolate bar		french fries

Tally your number for each column to determine
whether you favor sweet or non-sweet carbs.

of carbohydrate we are consuming, the impact that it has inside our bodies is relatively the same. Whenever we consume a carbohydrate-rich food choice, digestion takes place until glucose (sugar) units result. When excessive amounts of sugar are absorbed in the body, the brain releases large amounts of the neurotransmitter dopamine. In other words, sugar activates the brain's reward system, which is why sugar is so addicting!

The brain is not specific as to where the glucose comes from. If you consume pasta or a baguette, glucose is still present and can activate the brain's reward system—giving you that increased pleasure from dopamine. It's important to note that although carbohydrate choices such as bread and pasta may not seem like they contain high amounts of added sugars, oftentimes they do—which is why they can be difficult to resist! For example, one regular-sized plain bagel contains roughly 55 g of carbohydrates and about 9 g of added sugar! In other words, consuming one plain bagel at breakfast with no toppings is already 36 percent of your total added sugar intake for the day! If you add 2 tablespoons of flavored cream cheese or another topping, you may be even close to 50 percent of your total recommended intake.

The reason for sharing this information is to highlight that giving up carbohydrates isn't necessarily the solution to your intense cravings. Cutting back on pizza and bagels may not prove to be very effective in the long run. Instead, it's best to focus on cutting back on added sugars. Many processed foods contain simple carbohydrates in the form of added sugars, and these types of carbohydrates can be absorbed very quickly. The goal here is not to cut out carbohydrates entirely, but rather to reduce the sweetness of foods. From birth, we are born with sensory desires for sweeter foods, making food choices with added sugars more appealing to the brain. Restricting the intake of added sugars in the diet can decrease the cravings that arise for even non-sugary carbohydrate choices.

This book is focused on breaking your addiction to *added* sugar, the sweet stuff. But what should you do if you find that you're a total carb junkie and many of them (sweet or not) trigger you to overeat? Don't worry. You have to start someplace, and the best thing is to start working on cutting back on *added* sugars first and see how that impacts how you feel. You will soon find that kicking the added sugar will make it a lot easier for you to manage your intake of other carbohydrates.

What's the difference between the different types of sugar out there? Is one worse than the other? Warning: the sugar conversation can get confusing, very quickly. But don't worry—I'm going to sift through the jargon and get right to the point for you. This isn't going to be a biochemistry lesson, but it's important to cover some of the basics regarding sugars and carbohydrates, as this background information will be important for you to keep in mind as you start to think about the kinds of foods you like to eat and the addiction-like behaviors that might be leading you to overeat. Plus, this information will be helpful to keep in the back of your mind for when we get to chapter 3, where I'll discuss sugar addiction, as thinking about how different types of sugars impact your brain and body can help you to better understand why you may *feel* a certain way after you eat them.

The discussion of sugars could go on and on. We could talk about the glycemic index of sugars (some are high, others low) or the breakdown of "simple" versus "complex" carbohydrates. This type of information is great to know, but I don't think it helps much when trying to figure out how to cut sugar out of your diet. Here's why: if you get caught up with counting carbs, or trying to figure out if certain foods are "too high" or "too low" in terms of their glycemic index (which, by the way, is a generalization—how foods affect your blood sugar is unique to *your* body and health status, and even the time of day!), it quickly gets cumbersome and confusing. For example, a cup of cooked quinoa is 70 percent carbohydrates, but it's also a good protein source. So, do you eat it or not? Same with a banana. A large one can have 31 g of carbs. On the other hand, cheese sticks and pork rinds have 0 carbs, but are they healthy? I know there are lots of opinions out there, but anyone who tells you eating pork rinds instead of a banana is a healthy choice is just wrong.

The bottom line: There are too many shades of gray with counting carbohydrates or trying to figure out which carbs you should or shouldn't eat, leaving too much room for error and frustration. My advice is simple: forget the carb conversation and just work on reducing or avoiding the added sugars.

Okay, now that we have these questions squared away, let's talk about sugar.

A Sugar by Any Other Name Is . . . Still Sugar

The first step in this process is being able to identify sugar. But that isn't as easy as it sounds. Sugar isn't just sugar—it goes by more than 250 other names (see the Appendix on p. 269 for a list of them all)!

Some of the more common ones are shown in the sidebar on page 50. It's a good idea to familiarize yourself with this list, so that when you're looking at food labels you can recognize added sugars. Thanks to marketing tricks, many of these sugars don't even sound like sugar. Some of them are obviously sweeteners but sound like they are healthier for us (like agave nectar, or honey), while others don't even remotely sound like something that could be a sugar (like dextrin, maltol, or treacle).

Why are there so many different sugars out there? It wasn't always the case. Sugar in our foods used to just be in the form of sucrose that came from sugarcane or sugar beets. Then, thanks to advances in food technology, other sugars began to appear. Scientists started mixing and matching different forms of sugar. Part of it, more recently, has been because sugar has gotten a bad rap. Food companies need to sweeten food, but labeling a product as "fruit-juice sweetened" or "50% less sugar" sounds a lot better than having sugar listed as the primary ingredient. Also, companies have realized that they can add a bunch of sugars that have different names, and

NOT ALL CARBS ARE CREATED EQUAL

Just because something is "high carb" doesn't necessarily mean that it's unhealthy. Check out these examples of high-carb foods and compare them to less healthy low-carb options. Bottom line: it's the *added sugar*, not the carbs, that you should be considering!

High Carb		*Low Carb*
beets		beef jerky
black-eyed peas		heavy cream
squash		butter
sweet potatoes	VS	Coke Zero®
apples		ranch dressing
peas		high-fat cheese
corn		whipped cream
mangoes		pepperoni
bananas		pork rinds

COMMON NAMES FOR ADDED SUGARS

1. Sugar
2. High-fructose corn syrup
3. Sucrose
4. Fruit juice concentrate
5. Sorghum syrup
6. Corn syrup
7. Agave nectar
8. Raw sugar
9. Malt syrup
10. Cane sugar
11. Dextrose
12. Invert sugar

people won't necessarily realize that the product has a lot of added sugar. So if you pick up a product and the ingredients list includes agave syrup, fruit juice concentrate, sorghum molasses, and dextrin, someone none the wiser might assume that the product is sugar-free because the word *sugar* never appears. But in reality, this product contains four different forms of sugar!

Another reason is that not all sugars are exactly alike in how sweet they taste. There is a range of sweetness, and fructose (a sugar that naturally occurs in fruit) is the sweetest—it is almost two times as sweet as sucrose. Also, many different forms of sugar arise throughout the production process. For example, if you take sugarcane at various points along the line of how it is processed, you'll end up with cane sugar, evaporated cane sugar, raw sugar, brown sugar, turbinado sugar, blackstrap molasses, caster sugar, confectioners' sugar, and invert sugar—just to name a few. Some of these sugars have unique attributes that make them more or less desirable when baking or cooking. But at the end of the day, they are all just versions of sugar.

Figuring Out Fructose

Fructose is a sugar that can naturally be found in fruits, so one would think that makes it healthy, right? Not exactly. While consuming fruits (fruits naturally contain the sugars fructose and glucose in different amounts depending on the fruit) is a great idea, when you strip the fruit down and isolate just the fructose component, things can get ugly.

Excessive amounts of fructose can end up being stored as fat in our liver and cause the liver to be inflamed. As a result, people are more and more often developing diet-related fatty liver disease. Even kids are developing it. One in ten children has fatty liver disease. And that number has doubled over the past twenty years. Fatty liver disease used to be something that was most often seen in adults, and most often it resulted from being an alcoholic. But nowadays, diet is causing it (and has led to the creation of a new condition known as nonalcoholic fatty liver disease).

Does this mean you should limit your fruit intake? Absolutely not! The reason why fructose is causing liver problems for some individuals has *nothing* to do with eating fruit: the problem is when fructose becomes highly concentrated, as in the case of juices and sugars like high-fructose corn syrup.

STEALTHY (NOT "HEALTHY") SUGARS

It's purely due to marketing that many people think that when sugar isn't snow white, it's somehow better for you. Shoppers often pick up brown sugar or raw sugar thinking they are less refined than white (table) sugar, making them healthier. Not true. They are still highly processed and refined. In fact, brown sugar is often simply a combination of white sugar and molasses! Two sugars combined are definitely not better than one. Think about what you would need to do to go from a sugar beet that grows underground to a bag of crystallized brown sugar. It's a pretty big leap, and not exactly as *natural* as it is purported to be.

The same holds true for unrefined sugars like honey and agave—they are still sugar. And just because they come from nature doesn't mean that they are magically better for you. Lots of things come from nature that aren't good for you (poison mushrooms, mosquitoes, poison ivy, cocaine, etc.). Also, keep in mind that in actual nature, you would have to consume an awful lot of an agave plant to get the amount of sugar that you would get from a few squirts from a bottle of it that you buy at the store.

Move Over, Sugar, Here Comes High-Fructose Corn Syrup

Big Food is a part of this story. Fructose is sweeter than glucose or sucrose, meaning that food producers can add less of it to their product but get more sweetness for their money.

High-fructose corn syrup (HFCS) is the most well-known fructose sweetener that the food companies have used. HFCS comes from corn and found its way into the American food system in the early 1970s amid rising food prices and the unpredictable nature of sugar imports. Around this time, sugar prices were going up, and it was cheaper to make HFCS here in the US. By 1984, the major beverage makers, Coca-Cola® and Pepsi®, reformulated their products to swap out sugar for HFCS. HFCS was cheaper, shelf stable, and helped to improve the texture and taste of baked goods. Seemed too good to be true for both the food industry and the consumer. And guess what? It was.

For a while, food scientists argued that HFCS and sucrose were biologically identical. Sucrose is a disaccharide—this simply means it is made up of a glucose and a fructose molecule that are bonded together. HFCS is also a combination of glucose and fructose, but without the bond. We know for sure that sucrose contains glucose and fructose in equal proportions because the sugar molecules are paired up and are physically connected. But the problem with HFCS was that no one knew *for sure* how much glucose and fructose was included in the formulation. This is because food companies aren't required by law to disclose the amounts. They just have to list HFCS as an ingredient. So, when you eat a product containing HFCS, you have no way of knowing if the product contains HFCS-55 (which is 55 percent fructose) or HFCS-90 (which is 90 percent fructose), or one of the other several HFCS formulations that are out there.

In 2004, a well-known obesity researcher named Dr. George Bray published a paper that raised some red flags about HFCS. He showed there was an interesting correlation between the rise in obesity rates over time and the amount of HFCS that was being consumed by Americans. Correlation means that there is a relationship, but it doesn't necessarily mean that it's the cause. After reading Bray's paper, I became interested in studying this so we could better understand HFCS. If it's in so many things we eat, shouldn't we know exactly what it does to our bodies?

Shortly thereafter, my lab conducted some experiments looking at HFCS and sucrose. We found in our lab rats that those who were given HFCS to drink gained *significantly* more body weight than rats given equal access to a sucrose solution, even though they consumed the same number of total calories. We also looked at the long-term effects of HFCS on body weight and some parameters related to obesity and metabolic health. Over the course of six or seven months, both male and female rats with access to HFCS gained significantly more body weight than the control groups. This increase in body weight with HFCS was accompanied by an increase in adipose fat, notably in the abdominal region, as well as elevated circulating triglyceride levels.

We got a lot of pushback from the Corn Refiners Association on this after we published the paper. They immediately trashed the studies in the media, calling it "junk science" and saying the findings didn't matter because the study was conducted "in rats." But, very soon thereafter, others in the field started publishing clinical results from studies looking at HFCS. In one now well-known study often referred to as "the Dr Pepper® study," adults were given (you guessed it) Dr Pepper® to drink that was sweetened with either HFCS or sucrose; the results showed that there was 20 percent more fructose circulating in the blood after consuming HFCS-sweetened Dr Pepper® compared to sucrose-sweetened Dr Pepper®. Blood pressure and other markers for diabetes and cardiovascular disease were also

SPOTTING SUGAR: TIPS TO IDENTIFY ADDED SUGARS IN FOOD

- ends in -ose, it's a sugar
- has syrup in the name, it's a sugar
- has molasses in the name, it's a sugar

elevated after consuming HFCS-sweetened Dr Pepper® compared to sucrose-sweetened Dr Pepper®. Clearly, in rats and humans, HFCS and sucrose weren't the same.

KNOW YOUR NUTRITION FACTS LABEL

Chips Ahoy®

Nutrition Facts

about 11 servings per container
Serving size 3 cookies (33g)

Amount per serving

Calories 160

	% Daily Value*
Total Fat 8g	**10%**
Saturated Fat 2.5g	**13%**
Trans Fat 0g	
Cholesterol 0mg	**0%**
Sodium 110mg	**5%**
Total Carbohydrate 22g	**8%**
Dietary Fiber Less than 1g	**3%**
Total Sugars 11g	
Includes 11g Added Sugars	**22%**
Protein 1g	
Vitamin D 0mcg	0%
Calcium 5mg	0%
Iron 1.1mg	6%
Potassium 0mg	0%

*The % Daily Value (DV) tells you how much a nutrient in a serving of food contributes to a daily diet. 2,000 calories a day is used for general nutrition advice.

A serving size is a portion of food as recommended by the FDA.

→ Calories (units of energy) per serving.

→ The unhealthy type of fat, where eating too much can raise LDL cholesterol and greaten the chance of heart disease and stroke.

→ Sugars added during processing or preparation are considered "added" sugars. Consuming too many added sugars can increase risk of type II diabetes, heart disease, and other health conditions.

* Visit www.fda.gov for the most up-to-date nutritional information, including recommended daily value (%DV) for specific nutrients.

"Natural" Sugars and Why They Are Still Dangerous

HFCS isn't the only sugar out there that has excess fructose in it. Lots of sweeteners on the market that are perceived to be healthier than sucrose or HFCS because their names sound more natural, like fruit juice concentrate or agave, can actually have more fructose in them than HFCS. Agave syrup can contain up to 90 percent fructose. Also, fruit concentrates are often used to sweeten products, and many times people see "fruit" and think that it's good for them because it's derived from fruit. But when you "concentrate" fruit, you're taking away all of the fiber and many of the healthy vitamins, like vitamin C, and leaving behind just the sugar. When you see something that contains "fruit concentrate," know that the only part of the fruit you are getting is the sugar.

Honey has been used as a sweetener for almost 10,000 years. In the past, it was believed to help treat diseases. In addition, it has significance in multiple religions, including Buddhism, Islam, Judaism, Hinduism, and Christianity. The healthy benefits of honey come from its antifungal, antiviral, and antibacterial qualities. Honey contains essential vitamins and minerals, such as choline and acetylcholine, while regular sugar does not. In contrast to the other alternative sweeteners, honey is not low-calorie compared to table sugar. One tablespoon of honey has 64 calories, which is more calories than you would get from one tablespoon of table sugar

(48 calories). Therefore, substituting honey for table sugar might lead to excessive energy intake, causing weight gain.

Maple syrup, like honey, is a natural alternative sweetener that does not come with a lower caloric intake. Made from the sap of maple trees, it is then boiled down into the sweet syrup that can be found on the shelves. Maple syrup has a high concentration of manganese and zinc. The presence of these minerals leads many to believe that it's a healthy alternative to table sugar. It has fewer calories than honey but is still slightly higher than table sugar. Therefore, like honey, replacing regular sugar with maple syrup will not have the weight-loss effect that is usually desired.

Also, the primary reason why these alternative sugars are no better for you than actual sugar is because your brain doesn't know the difference. The sweet taste is what's driving your addiction. More on that in chapter 3.

Watch Out for "Healthy" Foods That Are Surprisingly High in Added Sugars

The challenge most of us face is figuring out which foods have sugar in them so that we can limit or avoid them. With all of the different names for sugar, and the fact that the food industry is sneaky with sugar and doesn't always make it clear that a product contains it, you have to do your homework and know what to look out for. Let's talk about some food categories where sugar can sneak its way in, and lower-sugar alternatives in these categories that you can try instead.

These may contain alternative sweeteners—and that is okay! If you're starting to cut down on your sugar intake, alternative sweeteners like monk fruit, stevia, and others may help, but be sure to see the sections later in the chapter about how the goal is to ultimately un-sweeten your diet, including reducing the use of these alternative sweeteners, too.

Breakfast Cereal

Many of the breakfast cereals you find in the grocery store advertise themselves as a "healthy" breakfast option. They may advertise the use of whole grains and the quality of the ingredients the cereal contains to back up that "healthy" claim. While this could be true, they neglect to highlight the fact that these cereals may also be high in sugar despite their other nutrient claims.

Consider Kellogg's® Special K® Fruit & Yogurt Cereal. One serving delivers 13 g of added sugar, and that's without including your choice of milk! Yikes! That's 26 percent of the daily recommended amount (just over a quarter of a day's worth of added sugar).

Instead opt for Quaker Life® or Honey Bunches of Oats®, which each contain only 6 g of sugar per serving. Kashi® Cinnamon French Toast (6 g of sugar per serving) and Original Cheerios® (1 g of sugar per serving) are lower-sugar options as well.

Bars

Bars are often sought after as an on-the-go snack to keep us full until our next meal. Not all bars are created equal. Some are considerably higher in sugar and lower in ingredients that will help to make you feel full, like protein.

A perfect example is the classic Chocolate Chip CLIF Bar®. This bar contains 17 g of added sugar (32 percent of the daily recommended amount).

Instead opt for KIND® bars (their Dark Chocolate Nuts & Sea Salt flavor contains only 5 g of sugar). Another lower sugar option is RXBAR®. While these bars contain around 13 g of sugar, they are sweetened with dates and contain no added sugars. They also contain 12 g of protein to keep you full throughout the day!

Greek Yogurt

Greek yogurt is an easy protein staple that provides a great source of calcium and probiotics for gut health. There are many kinds of yogurts out there to navigate, and you want to choose one that will provide the most bang for your buck. However, many popular brands of Greek yogurts that are flavored are riddled with added sugars. Carefully consider the sugar content of your yogurt when shopping or choose a plain version and add berries to sweeten it.

Yoplait® Strawberry Greek Whips!® Yogurt contains 10 g of added sugar per serving. That's equivalent to about 2 full teaspoons of sugar for one small cup of Greek yogurt.

Instead opt for FAGE® Total 5% Whole Milk Greek Yogurt, which has zero added sugar and 14 g of protein.

Flavored Coffee

Coffee has evolved from the average black cup of joe to a variety of types, flavors, and beverage sizes. Starbucks® is a known hot spot for coffee lovers, but its beverages can come with an excessive amount of added sugar. It isn't just Starbucks®—other coffee places have similar drinks that will also give you way more sugar than you need.

A grande Starbucks® Caramel Macchiato can house 33 g of added sugar per serving.

Instead opt for unsweetened coffee, tea, or espresso, and add some of your favorite (no-sugar-added) milk.

Pressed Juices

The produce section at the grocery store has its wall of fruit and vegetable juices readily available for you to purchase. These juices are advertised as containing a day's worth of nutrients from those foods, making them even more desirable. However, as discussed earlier, when you take just the juice, you're removing all of the fiber and many other nutrients and leaving behind sugar.

The Naked® brand Green Machine juice is advertised as the ideal healthy beverage to increase your fruit and vegetable consumption, yet they do not advertise the 53 g of total sugar per serving. This is where things can get tricky. In this example, there is no added sugar, but if you look at the label you'll see that the product is mostly fruit juice. Fruit juice doesn't "count" as being an added sugar according to the FDA. In this product, they boast there is juice (sugar) from 2¾ apples, ⅓ of a mango, ¹⁄₁₂ of a pineapple, ⅓ of a kiwi, and ½ a banana, along with several other ingredients, like grasses, kale, broccoli, and spinach. All juiced down and packaged for you in one convenient bottle. I am not discounting the health benefits of these ingredients, but they are better for you in their whole form, where you get the fiber and other nutrients. Plus, think about it. If you sat down to *eat* all the things listed above, how long would it take you, and could you even finish it all in one sitting? Eating them all would still provide you with the same amount of sugar (if you could finish it all), but over a longer period of time, and with the fiber to lessen the jolt of sugar to your brain. I'll talk more about eating versus drinking later in chapter 5, but for now just keep in mind that when you drink something it affects your brain, and satiety levels, very differently from when you eat something.

The bottom line: Be careful about beverages that contain fruit juices. Even though they aren't technically added sugars, you should treat them as such. Instead opt for Suja Uber Greens® fruit and vegetable juice, which contains only 5 g of sugar and 0 g of added sugar per serving.

Granola

Whether you're adding granola to your yogurt or eating it as a snack, you may be consuming more sugar than you realize. Yes, granola can be a source of whole grains, but if it's full of sugar it may be worth reconsidering.

Nature Valley® Oats and Honey Protein Granola contains 15 g of added sugar per ⅔ cup serving.

Instead opt for Purely Elizabeth® Organic Original Ancient Grains Granola, which contains 7 g of sugar per serving. It also has 2 g of fiber and 3 g of protein per serving, so it's filling while having fewer calories than many other brands. The Fit V'Nilla Almond granola by Bear Naked® is another great option that contains 4 g of sugar, 3 g of fiber, and 3 g of protein per serving.

Dried Fruit

Dried fruit is denser than fresh fruit, as the water has been removed during the dehydration process. The fruit may be processed with sugar to enhance the taste. Dried fruit can be a good option, but look at the labels to make sure that it doesn't contain added sugars.

Ocean Spray® Craisins contains 26 g of *added* sugar per ¼ cup (that's 52 percent of the daily recommended amount).

Instead opt for Ocean Spray® 50% Less Sugar Craisins, which contain only 12 g of sugar per ¼ cup serving. Additionally, dried apricots are a good choice when you want a low-sugar alternative to other dried fruits. Crispy Fruit snacks by Crispy Green® are also a great freeze-dried fruit with no added sugars.

Frozen Pizza

Frozen pizza is a popular quick dinner option for many families. Pizza can contain a high amount of sodium and fat, which isn't surprising, but what you may not know is that it can also contain a lot of added sugar.

DiGiorno® Rising Crust Frozen Pepperoni Pizza has 36 g of sugar per whole pizza, with over half of that coming from added sugars.

Instead opt for Amy's® Margherita Pizza with only 4 g of sugar per serving (12 g per whole pizza). California Pizza Kitchen® Thin Crust Margherita Pizza is another low-sugar option that also has only 4 g of sugar per serving (12 g per whole pizza).

Sports Drinks

Flavored water and sports beverages are more common now than ever. Sports beverages are made to enhance hydration during sport, but many people consume them outside of sport. Take Strawberry Banana BodyArmor®, for example, which contains 21 g of added sugar per serving. Instead opt for Nooma® Organic Sports Drinks, which have only 5 g of sugar and 0 g of added sugar, as it uses natural fruit extracts for flavor and stevia for sweetness. Additionally, Gatorade® Zero or Powerade® Zero are 0 sugar, 0 calorie alternatives to the sugar-packed Original Gatorade® drinks.

What Makes You Feel Full?

Feeling full, otherwise known as satiety, involves some interesting biological factors. You start to feel full from the chemicals that are released in your digestive tract when you eat or drink. But it isn't solely the result of the food or drink you consumed; a variety of different factors, including chewing and the time it takes you to consume meals, impacts your ability to feel full. Satiety also determines when you eat. If you feel satiated, you won't desire a snack before your next meal. Therefore, you'll have longer periods between eating. If you're not satiated, you'll look for something to fill your stomach. Therefore, you'll have shorter periods between eating.

However, not every food produces the same amount of satiety. Foods high in fiber and protein produce the highest level of satiety. High-protein foods such as meat, poultry, fish, and eggs are high-satiety foods. Foods rich in fiber, such as whole grains, legumes, fruits, and vegetables are also high in satiety. These foods will keep you fuller for longer, prolonging the time between eating. Fats and carbohydrates, on the other hand, produce less satiety. Therefore, high-carbohydrate foods, such as soda, pasta, pizza, and grains, and high-fat foods, such as fried foods and baked goods, produce very little satiety. Since these foods produce little satiety, it will be a shorter amount of time until you desire your next snack or meal.

Satiety is also produced by cognitive and sensory signals. The sight, smell, and oral sensation of the food all influence the amount of satiety that is produced and how much is consumed.

Alternative Sweeteners—Sugar's Deceptive BFF

Avoiding added sugars is tough, but if you are mindful of the juices, and look at the label to check how much added sugar the item contains, it should be easier, right? Yes, but the story gets a bit complicated when we introduce sugar's best friend, alternative sweeteners.

Alternative sweeteners are also referred to as low-calorie or no-calorie sweeteners. I lump these into the same category as artificial sweeteners, since when it comes to addiction, they are all the same. These sweeteners have been praised for decreasing caloric intake in particular foods. It's a lot easier to consume low-calorie alternatives with the same taste than it is to reduce intake. Many believe that consuming these low-calorie alternatives will lead to long-term weight loss. However, that may not be the case. Despite the increase in noncaloric sweeteners, the obesity rates in America have continued to rise. Therefore, noncaloric sweeteners might not be the weight loss solution we once thought they were.

Multiple alternative sweeteners have gained popularity with both the public and food manufacturers. Popular low-calorie alternative sweeteners include stevia, monk fruit, allulose, and sugar alcohols. Let's take a deeper look at each of these, and then I'll tell you why I'm not a fan of them.

Stevia. Stevia is a sugar substitute 150 to 200 times sweeter than table sugar. Only a small quantity is needed to provide the same sweetness as typical sugar, which means there will be fewer calories coming from the sweetener.

Monk Fruit. Monk fruit sweetener is another calorie-free sweetener. It comes from the juice of the monk fruit after the seeds and skin have been removed. Monk fruit sweetener contains zero calories per serving and is 150 to 200 times sweeter than table sugar. It is commonly used in baked goods since it is stable at high temperatures.

Allulose. D-allulose is found naturally in wheat, cane molasses, and itea plants. Used as a low-calorie sweetener, it is 70 percent as sweet as sucrose, but only has 0.4 calories per gram. It is commonly used in foods and drinks as it has no bitter aftertaste and can improve food gelling behavior. It also is highly active during the Maillard reaction, which gives cakes and cookies their brown color. Therefore, it is often utilized in baked goods and brown drinks.

Sugar alcohols. Sugar alcohols are a very popular alternative sweetener. They are made from sugar molecules but substitute a hydroxyl group on the molecule. As a result, they are very hard to digest and are not completely absorbed. Since they are not completely absorbed, they're considered lower in calories. However, given that they are hard to digest, they're known to have a laxative effect and can cause digestion problems, such as bloating and abdominal discomfort.

There are multiple types of sugar alcohols, each different based on the original sugar molecule it came from. Sorbitol, mannitol, isomalt, maltitol, lactitol, xylitol, and erythritol are the sugar alcohols that are used in food products. Sorbitol is used in a wide variety of products, including chewing gum, baked goods, frozen desserts, and sugar-free candies. Mannitol is found mainly in pharmaceutical and nutritional tablets. Isomalt is used in hard candies, toffees, chocolate, baked goods,

THE TRUTH ABOUT ERYTHRITOL

Research out of the Cleveland Clinic showed a correlation between erythritol levels in the blood and poor cardiovascular outcomes, which are similar consequences to what scientists have found regarding real sugar. The research looked at erythritol in particular (while not analyzing other sugar alcohols) and found a higher associated risk of thrombosis and major adverse cardiac event rates related to erythritol. So, should you ditch it?

More research is needed to know whether erythritol (and other sugar alcohols) could be deleterious to heart health. While sugar alcohols can be a useful tool to quit sugar, they should not be a crutch. Don't rely on chemical compounds to trick your brain into thinking you are still consuming sugar without the calories or weight gain. This will save your sanity and your heart! The recipes included in this book (see pp. 214–268) avoid alternative sweeteners altogether.

nutritional supplements, cough drops, and gum. Maltitol can be used as a fat substitute and is used in many baked products. Lactitol is typically combined with other low-calorie sweeteners and used in diet-based foods, such as low-calorie, low-fat, or sugar-free ice creams, chocolate, hard and soft candies, baked goods, and sugar substitutes. Since xylitol is the sweetest, it is a common ingredient in food, pharmaceutical, and nutraceutical products, including gum and candy. Erythritol is used in chewing gum, candy products, and ice cream.

The Problem with Alternative Sweeteners

There is some evidence to support that alternative sweeteners can reduce calorie intake in the short term. In one study, thirty-one individuals were given a preloaded sweetened beverage made either from stevia, aspartame (a noncaloric sweetener), or sucrose (table sugar) before eating a meal. The study found that people consumed the same amount of food at the meal regardless of what they drank beforehand. While the calories consumed at the meal were the same, the calories in the drinks were different. Since the noncaloric sweetener was lower in calories, the meals with the low-calorie beverage were lower in calories.

While this finding supports the belief that alternative/artificial sweeteners reduce caloric intake, the short-term caloric decrease might result in overeating in the long term. Animal studies have shown that stripping the calories from something that tastes sweet disrupts the animal's ability to regulate energy intake. In one study, rats that consumed saccharin-sweetened yogurt increased their intake of food. As a result, the rats gained weight and body fat. Artificial sweeteners causing overweight and obesity were also observed in humans. An analysis of several research studies found that in a group of cohort studies, low-calorie sweetener intake was positively associated with a higher BMI.

Multiple theories have evolved to explain why sweeteners that are lower in calories can cause weight gain. One explanation is that artificial sweeteners cause one's body to prefer sweet-tasting items. An animal study done on rats tested this theory. The rats were given either an artificially sweetened beverage or water for several days. They were then given two flavors. Both flavors were equal in calories, but one had a sweet taste and the other did not. If the rats preferred the sweeter beverage, it showed that the artificial sweetener preempted their body to prefer sweet things. However, if there was equal preference between the two drinks, it showed that the rats' preference for food was related to the caloric content of the food, not the flavor. The study found that the rats who were given the artificial sweetener preferred the sweetened beverage, confirming the idea that artificial sweeteners enhance the desire for sweet taste. The heightened preference for sweetness just adds fuel to the addiction fire and can result in overindulgence in sugar-sweetened foods, which are typically higher in calories.

Another theory behind low-calorie sweeteners causing weight gain is that they change the body's hormonal response to sweets.

Like regular sugar, artificial sweeteners activate the sweet taste receptor on the tongue and send the signal to the brain, particularly the
hypothalamus and amygdala. This process causes the feeling of satisfaction and reward that is normally associated with a sweet taste.
However, artificial sweeteners do not cause the same rise in blood
glucose and insulin that typically occurs with sugar. As a result, the
post-ingestion pathway is not activated, leading to increased appetite,
food cravings, and caloric consumption.

Rodent studies have also found that consuming artificial sweeteners affects the release of GLP-1, the hormone responsible for
controlling appetite suppression and satiety signaling. A study tested
the response rats had to sugar after being fed artificial sweeteners.
The rats had hyperglycemia. This meant they had a high level of
sugar in their blood, suggesting their body wasn't properly handling
the sugar intake. The same study also showed that the rats had a
decreased thermogenic effect of food. Therefore, the body is burning fewer calories when it is digesting food. Finally, the study showed
that the rats had decreased satiety and increased caloric intake. All
of these effects can lead to weight gain and obesity.

Lastly and most importantly, as I mentioned earlier, when you
use these alternative sweeteners, your brain doesn't know that it's
fake. It thinks it's real sugar. I'll go into this in greater detail in
chapter 3, where I'll talk about addiction, but it's the sweet taste
that is driving the addiction to sugar, and when the taste of any of
these sweeteners hits your tongue, the message gets sent to your

brain that you are tasting something sweet, feeding into the sugar addiction cycle.

Bottom line: Alternative sweeteners can be a crutch if you're trying to get off real sugars, but to really be able to heal your brain and get free from your addiction, the ultimate goal should be to reduce added sweeteners in your diet. I view them like methadone: it's better for you than heroin and can help when you're trying to detox, but you don't want to stay on it forever.

Now that you know how to find sugar in your food, and all the ways that it can sneak in, the next step is to deal with how to break your addiction to it. But first, let's talk about what addiction means, and how sugar fits in.

SUGAR IS ADDICTIVE

I remember being a kid in the 1980s and seeing for the first time the public service commercial warning against drug use. A guy held up an egg and said, "This is your brain"; then the camera panned to a sizzling frying pan, and he said, "This is drugs." Then he cracked the egg into the pan and said, "This is your brain on drugs. Any questions?" I was probably eight or nine years old the first time I saw that commercial, but looking back, that simple yet effective message had a significant impact on me. Not only did it scare me away from ever trying drugs (the thought of my brain sizzling like an egg was enough to scare me away from even *thinking* about trying them), but it probably also contributed to me eventually studying the brain.

This commercial from the 1980s came out during the cocaine addiction crisis that was happening in the US at the time. In response to the sudden increase in addiction and overdoses, the US launched the "War on Drugs," an anti-drug effort to combat illegal drug use. Back then, addiction was solely synonymous with drugs and alcohol. However, that is now changing, and research has shown that addiction is not limited to these few substances, and in fact can expand far beyond them. Doctors agree that people can become addicted to activities, such as gambling, video games, and sex—and even sugar. We are unfortunately still fighting the war on drugs and have added to that multiple parallel wars—a big one being the war on sugar.

How Addictions Develop

One of the difficult things to understand about substance abuse is that not everyone gets addicted. Some people can have a few glasses of wine now and then and be fine, while others can't stop. Same goes for smoking an occasional cigarette, or even using harder drugs recreationally. This is also the case with sugar—some people can stop at one cookie, while others find that they can't control themselves and end up eating more than they wanted to.

It's almost as if there's a switch point at which people cross over from engaging in a behavior, like drinking or eating, in a controlled manner because they enjoy it and get pleasure from it, to then suddenly being in a situation in which they no longer have control, and no longer really even get reward from it. Any little reward or joy that they do experience is quickly washed away by shame, guilt, and regret.

Addictions develop in response to repeated exposures, and changes in the way we process reward. In fact, scientists have developed a theory to describe how addictions develop; it's called the Opponent-Process Theory. When someone first uses a substance, they feel a "high," the reward from it, and a "low" after. But with repeated use, the highs get less intense, while the lows get more intense. It gets to the point where many people find they are using the substance to avoid the lows and just to try to feel like they are back at baseline or "normal" again.

Behaviors become addicting because of the way the brain responds to rewarding activities. Our brains are broken into regions that are responsible for controlling specific functions. Some regions are responsible for feeling pleasure, reward, and memory, while others are responsible for motivation and control. Each region works individually while also communicating with the other regions. To communicate between regions, the brain uses neurotransmitters. Neurotransmitters are chemical signals that travel to or stay away from certain regions of the brain in response to what is happening in the environment and our bodies.

For example, if we smell a fresh apple pie coming out of the oven, we recall what it tastes like, decide to have a piece, and walk over to grab a slice. For this to happen, neurotransmitters must activate certain pathways in the brain and the body. In this example, neurotransmitters must have played a role in activating the memory of the taste and motivating us to walk over and have a slice. After having a bite of the warm pie, neurotransmitters would also activate the systems responsible for feelings of reward and pleasure and tell us when to stop eating.

HOW ADDICTIONS DEVELOP

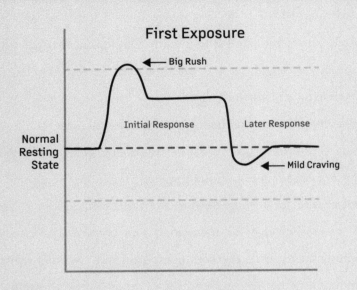

First Exposure

Big Rush

Initial Response

Later Response

Normal
Resting
State

Mild Craving

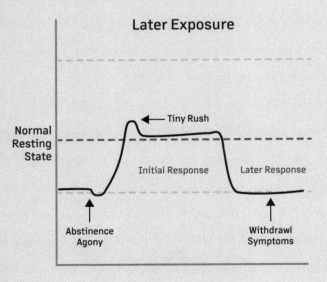

Later Exposure

Normal
Resting
State

Tiny Rush

Initial Response

Later Response

Abstinence
Agony

Withdrawl
Symptoms

However, the addicted brain has neurotransmitters that act differently from the nonaddicted brain. When a brain is addicted to drugs, specific neurotransmitters start to act differently in key regions, specifically the reward-related region, and this leads to people getting trapped in the spiral of bingeing, withdrawal, and craving that characterizes addiction.

Defining Addiction

It is very important that we have a clear definition of addiction, because if we are going to see whether sugar can meet the criteria for it, we need to have those criteria outlined. Most medical professionals view the American Psychiatric Associations Diagnostic and Statistical Manual of Mental Disorders (DSM) definition of addiction, or rather, for "substance-related and addictive disorders." There are presently eleven criteria, and meeting just one of them puts you at risk. If you meet two or three, you may have mild substance use disorder; if you meet four or five, moderate; and if you meet six or more, that is said to be an addiction. These criteria are shown in the figure, and on page 280 you can take a quiz that is based on these criteria to help you determine the extent of your addiction to sugar.

In addition to these behavioral criteria, there are changes in the brain that occur as one develops an addiction. Dopamine is a neurotransmitter that responds to pleasurable experiences, such as eating certain foods, having sex, or using drugs and alcohol. Dopamine plays a large role in reward-related regions. The pleasure that comes

CRITERIA FOR SUBSTANCE USE DISORDER

1. Tolerance

2. Withdrawal

3. Hazardous use

4. Social/interpersonal problems

5. Neglected major roles to use

6. Used larger amounts/longer

7. Attempts to quit/control use

8. Much time spent using

9. Physical/psychological problems

10. Activities given up to use

from rewarding experiences is derived from the release of dopamine. Therefore, it is the release of dopamine in response to these activities that makes them pleasurable. This system can go awry when it comes to addiction. When addicted, the dopamine response is altered, producing too many or too few feelings of reward in response to these activities. As a result, individuals become hooked on trying to capture the feeling of reward, resulting in their overindulgence in the substance or activity. They are always "chasing the high" that they recall getting from the drug, and never quite able to grasp it.

Here's the crazy part: the reward system that is activated by drugs and changed to make them addicting is the *same* system that is activated by the foods we eat. We don't have a cocaine system, or an alcohol system, or a cupcake system; it is all one system, a reward system. Our brain doesn't know if we are shooting heroin or eating a cupcake. This is why it makes sense that many of the foods we eat, especially the highly processed man-made foods that are loaded with added sugar, can be addictive—they affect the brain like a drug would.

Before I get into talking about the neuroscience research on sugar and how it affects the brain, let's start at the beginning and review some of the initial research studies that were conducted to allow us to test whether or not sugar addiction is real.

Characterizing Sugar Addiction

We started off doing research on sugar addiction using animal models. Rats and mice are commonly used in research settings since their brain systems and neural circuitry are similar to humans. In addition, rats don't care if they look good in a bikini. This means that by conducting research on rodents we can create a completely objective situation by reducing the risk of outside factors, such as self-esteem, environment, media, or culture, from affecting the results of a study. Therefore, rats are good models of the human brain in our response to certain stimuli, especially food.

To assess if addiction was present, we analyzed whether the rats presented some components of addiction: bingeing, withdrawal, and craving. Bingeing is defined as the escalated high intake of a substance at one time after a period of not consuming the substance. Withdrawal is defined as negative affect or anxious behaviors that occur when a substance is no longer available. Craving is defined as enhanced motivation to obtain a substance after a period of abstinence.

In the model we developed, rats were deprived of food for twelve hours and then given access to a sugar solution, water, and rat chow (which is a healthy, balanced diet for a rat—kind of like dog food but for rodents) for twelve hours. We chose twelve hours per day because we wanted to encourage the rats to binge on the sugar when they got it each day, but we also wanted it to be available for most of the time that they were awake (the majority of the time that they didn't have access to sugar was when they were sleeping). We also included control groups, so that we could understand if different patterns of amount of access to sugar could produce differed effects on behavior. We included groups that were allowed to drink sugar, plain water, and have food 24/7, and also a group that was allowed to have their food and water for just twelve hours per day (to control for any influence that having limited daily access to anything—even something healthy—might have).

After a month of being fed on these different diets, we conducted several different experiments and systematically began to look for signs of addiction. Study after study, we started to note something very interesting: the rats that had binge access to the sugar were in fact bingeing on it, and they were also showing other signs of addiction. They were escalating their intake each day (tolerance), and when we deprived them of the sugar for a few days, they showed signs of withdrawal. They also seemed to be craving it. Lastly, their brains had changed—when we looked at what was happening in terms of their neurotransmitters, the brains looked more like a rat that was hooked on drugs.

After our first few research studies were published in scientific journals, the research revolving around sugar addiction rapidly expanded. More scientists and clinical researchers began wondering about the addictive nature of sugar and other foods—and this became a new area of inquiry. Importantly, the first clinical characterization of food addiction came a few years after we began our rodent studies. Food addiction was first operationalized using the Yale Food Addiction Scale (YFAS), which adapts the American Psychiatric Association's diagnostic criteria for substance use disorders to reflect an addictive-like response to certain foods. Using this scale, it was found that food addiction was detected in many individuals, and certain factors, like increased body weight and a history of binge eating, increased the odds of one meeting the criteria for having an addiction. And, no surprise to you I'm sure, guess what the common denominator was in the foods that many people felt addicted to? *Added sugar.*

Let's look a bit more closely at the evidence that exists for each of these elements of addiction—bingeing, withdrawal, and craving—so that in chapter 4, we can begin the work of reversing this course and lessening your dependence on added sugars. There are so many studies on this topic that I can't possibly cover them all in this chapter, so I'll highlight the main topics, and in the references section I have noted many more studies that are relevant to the development of the field.

Sugar Bingeing and Tolerance

Bingeing (taking in more than intended) and tolerance are two criteria for addiction. We showed in our early model that when offered sugar, rats will binge on it. They also consumed more and more each day, which suggests they were developing tolerance to it. Clinical research has shown that humans will engage in bingeing behavior, particularly on sweets. Much of the research conducted around binge eating considers this type of behavior as criteria for an eating disorder (and Binge Eating Disorder is recognized in the most recent edition of the DSM); however, the factors that lead to a binge are complex, and bingeing behavior can occur in individuals who do not necessarily meet the diagnostic criteria for an eating disorder. In fact, 5 percent of US adults engage in binge eating regularly. In addition, studies have revealed that certain situations, like stress, can precipitate binge eating. During a binge, one can feel euphoric, but this feeling is fleeting and often followed by feelings of guilt and shame. Over time, the consequences of repeated binges are associated with increased frequency of body weight fluctuation, depression, anxiety, and even abuse of other substances such as drugs and alcohol.

So what is keeping people in the cycle of consuming excess amounts of sugar and bingeing on it? Simply put, those who are bingeing on sugars build up tolerance. Tolerance is the threshold at which you feel the effects of a substance. Those who have been bingeing for years physiologically need more sugar to feel the pleasurable effects they desire. The problem is that they never get there, and like a drug addict they are chasing a sugar high that is unattainable. Even though our rational brains know this, the primitive parts of our brains win out and cause us to continue to binge in the absence of any true reward. And to make matters worse, repeated bingeing can lead to another sign of addiction: withdrawal.

Addiction and Eating Disorders: Is There a Link?

Binge eating is a type of eating disorder, and while the concept of sugar addiction is most closely aligned with this condition, there are other eating disorders, including bulimia and anorexia, where addiction to food could be involved. However, most practitioners are averse to adopting an addiction model for the treatment of eating disorders. Why is this? Well, mostly it is because the traditional model for treating eating disorders has focused on the tenet that there are no "good or bad" foods and patients should learn to eat "all foods in moderation." I don't agree with this as a strategy to use across the board for two reasons: most of the problematic foods that people are addicted to are highly processed man-made concoctions, not "food" in my opinion, and these items are designed to make people overeat them. Why make someone think that they have to learn to eat junk food in moderation, when by just avoiding it they can improve their health? That said, some eating disorder patients struggle with obsessive healthy eating as a mode for restriction, so while this book emphasizes healthy eating as a lifestyle choice, it does not condone malnutrition, but rather promotes better nutrition based on scientific literature and research.

Sugar Withdrawal

Withdrawal is another criterion for addiction. The type of behaviors one might exhibit when in withdrawal vary depending on the type of drug and also the length of use. For example, if someone is battling a severe alcohol addiction, they can develop seizures when they stop using as a result of withdrawal, which is why in these cases withdrawal or detox needs to be medically supervised. On the other hand, if someone is extremely addicted to nicotine, their withdrawal wouldn't require hospitalization, but would be characterized by irritability, craving, nausea, or anxiety.

People who have been on the diet roller coaster know all too well about the reality of sugar withdrawal. If you've been eating a diet high in added sugar and processed foods, and you make an abrupt change (like on New Year's Day, when many vow to clean up their diet), you might feel good for a few days, but then suddenly you feel like crap. Your symptoms include irritability, anxiety, lethargy, and headaches. Many people misattribute these feelings to their blood sugar dropping, and the cure for these negative feelings is, you guessed it, to eat something with sugar in it, which perpetuates the cycle of yo-yo dieting. But, in reality, the irritability, lethargy, headaches, and other symptoms are your brain's way of coping with the fact that you are no longer feeding it sugar and processed foods all of the time. This is sugar withdrawal.

For many years, reports of sugar withdrawal were anecdotal, but now the science supports this even more. Early in my research, I had a light-bulb moment about the reality of sugar withdrawal one afternoon when I was working in the lab. We had planned to see whether signs of withdrawal would emerge if we took the sugar away from the rats for a few days. Normally, lab rats are extremely docile and friendly, and you can pick them up and pet them. However, when, for one of our experiments, we took their sugar away for two days, that all changed. When I went in the animal room to weigh the rats and measure their food intake, the first one I picked up bit me! This was not at all normal. I let the little guy be and went on to the next rat. He, too, was agitated and squealed when I tried to pick him up. Again, this was not typical behavior! Turns out, this was a behavioral manifestation of their sugar withdrawal. As a side note, we never published the biting incident, but a few years later another group of researchers did, and noted the agitation as an indication of sugar withdrawal.

Many studies support that sugar withdrawal can develop. We first detected withdrawal from sugar in our rat studies when we removed sugar from rats that had been bingeing on it. After only twenty-four hours of no sugar, the rats showed signs that they were agitated and in a negative state—symptoms such as teeth clicking, tremors, and head shakes were observed. They were also found to be very anxious and had signs of behavioral depression or impulsivity in other studies.

Clinical studies have shown that in humans, individuals who consume highly processed foods—containing high amounts of sugar—may also experience symptoms of withdrawal. When assessing withdrawal in individuals who are experiencing food addiction, withdrawal has been reported by almost 55 percent of individuals (interesting, this is also found among children and adolescents, 56 percent of whom report withdrawal-like craving when they try to cut down on highly processed foods). Also, individuals who cut back on foods high in refined carbohydrates (i.e., sugars) through dieting efforts report withdrawal symptoms, such as headaches or fatigue. Paralleling the course of drug withdrawal, symptoms assessed for highly processed food withdrawal have been reported as most intense between days two through five during an attempt to cut down.

Altogether, these findings suggest that withdrawal signs *can* and *do* emerge in response to foods with added sugars. Does this sound all too familiar to you? Don't worry, we'll revisit the topic of sugar withdrawal in chapter 5, and I will give you some practical tips for how to get through it.

Sugar Craving

The term *cravings* can be described as an intense urge to eat a certain food. Cravings are a normal part of the appetitive process. We are supposed to have them. In many cases, they can signal to us that we are low on calories, or that we are deficient in a nutrient. For instance, if you're thinking about what to eat for dinner, and feel like having a hamburger, this could be because you're starting to be deficient in iron (and iron, among other nutrients, is found in beef, and if you have been eating beef in the past, your body has put this food-nutrient connection together). Cravings can be adaptive and protective.

However, the problematic cravings that many people encounter, and that often derail them from their sugarless goals, are not due to calorie or nutrient needs. Instead, these cravings are the result of *hedonic hunger*, or the desire to eat something simply due to the pleasurable sensations it provides. Sugar, for many of the neuroscientific reasons I will get into shortly, is the perfect way to satisfy hedonic pleasure seeking.

Food cravings are something that often leads to eating the very food you've been trying to avoid. Strong cravings associated with drugs and alcohol are directly related to relapse, which mirrors what you probably have experienced when trying to give up sugar. You try to avoid it, but if the sugar craving is too strong, willpower alone isn't enough to overcome it. Unfortunately, you probably aren't craving kale or other low-calorie foods, but more likely something sweet and calorically dense like chocolate cake or a candy bar. People don't crave bland food but favor highly palatable foods instead. Sometimes you might not be craving one particular food, but rather an assortment of candy or any sugary foods. Keep in mind that a food craving can even be for an entire food group or just food in general. There are also different reasons why we crave. One main reason is the food cues we are constantly bombarded with daily. You can't turn on the television or pass a billboard on the highway without seeing an ad for a high-sugar food. If you live in a big city, chances are you pass a fast-food establishment quite often. Commercials, print ads, the actual food itself, and the smell of the food are cues and have been shown to increase cravings.

Besides external food cues in our environment, you also must contend with internal food cues. Stress, hormonal changes, our thoughts, and our emotions can all contribute to food cravings. In research, food cravings can be measured subjectively by simply having people fill out questionnaires; however, cravings are so powerful that they can also be measured by a physical response. Your heart rate may go up and you might start salivating at the thought of eating your favorite chocolate brownie. Just seeing a picture of a chocolate bar not only increases the subjective craving for chocolate, it also leads to heightened responses in the brain.

As mentioned before, not all food cravings turn into much more than just giving in to sugar occasionally. However, if the cravings are persistent and always too hard to resist, they contribute to problematic eating behaviors, and sweets and certain carbs seem to have that negative effect. A recent study found that addictive-like eating behaviors and binge eating were partially mediated by cravings for sweets and other carbohydrates, suggesting that cravings for sugary foods can lead to pathological eating patterns.

Cravings for a particular substance also intensify the longer you abstain from it. This is seen in deadly drugs like heroin, as well as sugar. When rodents are given unlimited access to sugar and heroin and then forced to abstain, their drug- and sugar-seeking behaviors intensify. Unfortunately, over time, avoiding sugar might get harder before it gets easier, especially if you live or work in an environment where highly palatable foods are seemingly everywhere. You might be going about your day not planning on having any dessert, but since you passed the bakery on your lunchtime walk, you now find yourself craving a cookie. One large review study analyzing forty-five research papers found that seeing the food and the subsequent craving significantly influences eating behavior. This paper looked at data from over 3,000 participants, so take solace in the fact that you're not alone for indulging after seeing a tray of cookies in a bakery window.

If this happens too often, though, it can be problematic. Since sugar cravings typically lead to subsequent sugar intake, this can often lead to unintentional weight gain, which also plays a role in how our brain processes sweets. One study found that compared to women who were weight stable, those who gained weight over a six-month period had lower sensitivity in reward-related pathways in the brain when given a milkshake. This study supports the notion that weight gain may lead to decreased brain response to sweets, which can lead to needing more to get the same reward that one used to get from less. So instead of having one piece of cake to elicit a feel-good response, weight gain might lead to needing two pieces of cake for that same feeling. The part of the brain that showed less activation during the milkshake challenge is implicated not only in reward but in cravings too.

Another study found that people with obesity and food addiction showed a greater response in regions of the brain associated with craving when viewing pictures of highly palatable foods compared to those without food addiction. In addition, they exhibited lower response when viewing minimally processed foods in regions associated with cue-induced cravings.

Taken together, the reward-related regions of our brains respond to food and food cues in such a way that can make us crave more. Your own average weight status, any weight gain, prolonged abstinence, your daily food environment, and food cues all play a role in how the brain's reward regions respond to sugar and cravings, further complicating the matter. But luckily, more research continues to be done in this area.

As with the case of withdrawal, cravings are *real* and can be intense and sudden when it comes to foods with added sugars. If

SUGAR VS. COCAINE

Studies have also compared just how addicting sweet taste is compared to abusive drugs, such as cocaine. When rats are allowed to choose between sweetened water or intravenous cocaine, 94 percent of the animals choose sweetened water instead of cocaine, suggesting that the taste of sweetness can surpass cocaine reward.

you've been experiencing sugar cravings, and these have been a big factor in why you can't cut back on your sugar intake, don't worry. We'll come back to the topic of sugar cravings in chapter 5, and I will give you some practical tips for how to deal with them, and what to do to help prevent them from happening in the first place.

All of the behaviors that can come about from being addicted to drugs—the bingeing, withdrawal, anxiety, depression, and craving—are also now happening with sugar. Addiction is a vicious cycle—all these behaviors can feed off each other, creating anxiety that leads to cravings, which can lead to bingeing, which can lead to depression, and so on. And these behaviors aren't happening on their own. They are being fueled by, and are also at the same time fueling, the brain. An addicted brain acts very different from a nonaddicted one. Remember back in the beginning of this chapter when I talked about that old commercial, "This Is Your Brain on Drugs"? Well, folks, this is your brain on sugar. Let's now turn to the research on exactly how sugar messes with your brain.

The Addicted Brain

Dopamine is an important neurotransmitter in our brain. It has various functions, but one of them is that it plays a critical role in reward. In fact, dopamine release is the hallmark of drug use—each time a person smokes a cigarette, drinks alcohol, or uses heroin, dopamine is released in reward-related areas of the brain. When this happens, time after time, additional changes occur in the brain that make the individual crave the drug, contributing to the vicious spiral of addiction that can be extremely difficult to break out of.

Dopamine is often talked about for its role in addiction, but keep in mind that addiction is an extreme form of reinforcement. Dopamine also plays a role in reward and reinforcing behaviors that we *should* continue to do because they are good for us. Since we need food for our survival, it makes sense that eating food should be rewarding, especially when we are hungry. We need food to satisfy our basic survival needs, so our brains are designed to seek out and consume food when we are hungry. However, the brain responds to foods differently than it does to drugs and alcohol. Typically, dopamine is released when new, novel food is consumed. The release of dopamine is tied to our primitive nature as humans. When food was not guaranteed in our environment, our bodies had a drive to find and eat all the food we could when it was available. However, not all the food our ancestors found and consumed was safe. Therefore, to alert our ancestors of any new food, our brains would release dopamine. This alerted our ancestors that this was a new food and caused them to pay attention to how it tasted in case it made them sick later on.

This release of dopamine in response to new foods is still evident in our brains today. As foods become a staple in our diets and are deemed to be safe by our bodies, the dopamine response to the food decreases. Therefore, dopamine should only be released for new, risky eating behaviors, such as trying new foods. This is what originally differentiated the dopamine response between food and drug abuse: dopamine is released only during specific eating situations and decreased over time, while dopamine is *always* released after using a drug.

This is where added sugar and highly palatable foods become problematic. When you eat them in excess, your brain releases dopamine as if you are using a drug.

This Is Your Brain on Sugar

Our early studies of looking at the brains of sugar-addicted rats revealed some telling findings: their brains looked just like they were addicted to drugs, but the only drug they had access to was sugar.

As I mentioned above, dopamine release in reward-related brain regions is a hallmark of drug use, whereas foods don't typically release dopamine unless they are new. But when we looked at the brains of our rats that were hooked on sugar, they released dopamine every time they drank it. Even after multiple times drinking it. Just as if it was a drug. And not at all what we would have expected to see from a food. In fact, the control groups that were only having sugar once in a while didn't show this repeated release of dopamine. Their brains treated the sugar like a normal food, and the dopamine release attenuated after the initial exposure once the sugar didn't make the rats sick.

Next, we wanted to see whether the opposite would happen during withdrawal from sugar. Many research studies have shown that during withdrawal from drugs of abuse, like cocaine, nicotine, and morphine, the opposite happens to dopamine—it drops. And when we took sugar away from our bingeing rats, that is exactly what happened. This lack of dopamine explains, in part, some of the behaviors associated with withdrawal, such as anxiety and depression.

It is important to note that dopamine isn't the only neurotransmitter involved in this process. We have something known as the "endogenous opioid system," which plays a role in the pleasure response, and also helps to reduce feelings of pain. When you are injured, your brain releases opioids to help make you feel better. Opiate drugs (like heroin and morphine) are extremely addictive for this very reason. Studies show the endogenous opioids are altered when addicted to sugar, just like when someone is addicted to opiates.

This change in the brain's landscape and how it functions as a result of overeating sugar has been captured across many different human studies, as well. Using brain-scanning techniques, we have learned a lot about how the human brain responds to the thought, anticipation, or consumption of sugars.

Functional magnetic resonance imaging (fMRI) and positron emission tomography (PET) scans are painless, noninvasive ways to see how one's brain is functioning. fMRIs can measure the blood flow in the brain that helps indicate which part of the brain is activated. PET scans are similar, but rather use the activity of neurotransmitters to determine which brain region is being activated.

In one study utilizing fMRI, people with high food addiction scores who anticipated food had increased activation of the anterior cingulate cortex of the brain. This is the same area of the brain that is activated when cigarette smokers are exposed to smoking cues, such as a picture of a cigarette. In addition, PET scans have also found that obese individuals have less dopamine receptor availability, which is also found in individuals with drug addictions. This finding has been explained through the lens of a theory known as the reward deficiency syndrome, which argues that these individuals have a lower-functioning reward system and therefore must overindulge in rewarding activities, such as eating, to feel the same feeling of reward that others would feel.

Further, different foods have been shown to stimulate different areas of the brain. In one study, after consuming foods high in sugar, people had higher activation in the areas of the brain associated with regulating addictive behaviors than when they consumed foods such as vegetables. Therefore, it seems that the foods that are high in sugar can change the brain so that hunger and cravings are promoted, which over time can contribute to the development of an addiction.

Cue the Sugar

In addition to how our brains respond to high-sugar foods, we are constantly reminded to eat these foods. Not only are they ample in our environment, but we are being prompted to consume them on a nonstop basis. From advertisements popping up in your feed to shops on the side of a street, there are constant cues to consume these types of foods, leading to overconsumption. How does this happen? Believe it or not, even the *cues* associated with food can hijack your brain and lead you to want to eat more sugar.

We first studied this in our lab rats. We trained them to press a lever to get a sugar solution to drink. There is a light bulb above the lever, and whenever the bulb was illuminated, that meant that the rat would get the sugar if they pressed the lever. If the light bulb was off, no sugar was available. The rats came to associate the cue of the light bulb illuminating with the dispense of sugar solution when they pressed the lever. Rats are pretty smart—it didn't take long for them to figure this out.

After this association was established, the rats were denied sugar and its associated cue for at least thirty days, and their response rate was measured again after this time period had passed. We found that when addicted to sugar, the rats are more willing to press the lever to get sugar. They are willing to work harder, even for the cue that is associated with sugar. Other researchers have utilized a similar experimental design to demonstrate how environmental cues, when they have become associated with an addictive substance (sugar), result in a higher response rate from rats when presented with a cue, especially after the rats have abstained from ingesting the substance for a significant period. Now, I know these are rats we're talking about, but think about the human equivalent. If rats want a sugar substance when they see a light bulb that used to come on when sugar was available, what do you think your brain does when you see an ad for your favorite sweet snack, or walk past the ice-cream or coffee place that has your favorite sweet treat?

Rats are also "resistant to response extinction" when it comes to sugar. This is psychological jargon for the rats refusing to accept that there is no sugar available. Even when the light bulb is off (which means no sugar is available), rats who are addicted run over and start pressing the lever. They want the sugar so badly that even though they know there isn't any available, they keep trying for it anyway. Can you relate? Have you ever opened up your fridge or pantry and just stared in blankly?

Clinical studies have also demonstrated the power of food cues. In an experiment using elementary-age children compared to adults, researchers decided to expose the subjects to food advertisements on TV. They wanted to see if these kinds of exciting advertisements and marketing strategies led children to prefer different foods, and therefore overconsume them every time they saw the commercial. They found that when prompted by the TV to purchase or consume a specific food, the children were more likely to try and therefore enjoy that food. When we are cognitively occupied by other tasks, like working or cleaning the house, scientists found that our brains react subconsciously to food advertisement. Participants in a study that had a heavier cognitive load were 43 percent more likely to choose unhealthy food choices when listening to or watching TV commercials. This leads us to assume that not only does seeing advertisements for unhealthy foods lead us to over-consumption and poor diet choices, but also hearing it, even if we're not consciously paying attention to the content, stimulates a pathway in our brains telling us to eat! Our brains become programmed to crave these foods. When the demand gets so high, sugar addiction thrives. Think about how distracted we are these days, with smartphones and multitasking—it's no wonder that we're overeating sugar.

Unfortunately, dietary intake of excess sugar can lead to a vicious cycle of craving and overeating that can be stimulated by exposure to food cues, like an advertisement for a new brand of soda or candy bar. Research has shown that people who consume higher levels of sugar exhibit stronger responses in parts of their brain associated with reward and decision-making when exposed to food cues. Simultaneously, these individuals exhibited reduced blood levels of proteins responsible for satiety. This means that the mere exposure to a stimulus such as a billboard or commercial that advertises foods that typically activate reward pathways in the brain (sugary drinks and sweets) can ignite cravings that are hard to resist. The longer this pattern continues, the harder it is to break.

▶●◀

We covered a lot in this chapter, but I hope you now are convinced that there's a lot of research backing up what most of us have known all along: sugar can be addictive. Next, we are going to use this information to our advantage, and I'll show you how you can beat your addiction using psychology and neuroscience.

CHAPTER 4

BREAKING YOUR DEPENDENCE ON SUGAR

This is where the work (and the fun) begins.

You might be a little apprehensive at this point, as you have most likely been down this road of "starting the program" and implementing the "plan" many times before, and it didn't work. Or if it did work, it only worked for a while, and you slowly slid back to where you started. That's not going to happen this time, because this isn't that type of plan.

I am going to teach you how you can completely change your mindset around what you eat. You will no longer use food to soothe or reward yourself. You will no longer be a victim of the addiction machine that our modern food environment has created. I am going to show you how to break away and to use food for what it is intended to be: fuel for your body.

Let's look at an analogy. When you hit the gas station to fuel up your car, would you add diesel fuel if your car runs on gasoline? No! Or, if you have an electric car, would you put fuel in it instead of plugging it in to charge? No way! Why? Because your car wouldn't run correctly, and you would probably screw up the engine and cause yourself a bunch of problems (not to mention unnecessary costs). Even if diesel fuel were on sale, and easier to get quickly because there was no line, it still wouldn't make any sense to use it in these cases.

The same goes for food. You don't want to fill your tank with things you know won't allow you to function at your best. Even if sugar-rich processed food is cheaper and easier to get, in the long run, the costs to your health are greater. Think back to chapter 1 when we reviewed all the physical, cognitive, and mental health issues that are exacerbated by sugar. Then think back to chapter 3, when we learned how sugar can hijack your reward system, leading us to want more and more of it. Sugar is bad for you. You know it, and now you can do something about it.

I am going to teach you seven simple steps to break your addiction to sugar, but first, some ground rules.

Rule 1: There Is No Rush

The quick-fix mentality won't work here. In fact, it is that mentality that may have gotten you here in the first place. Everyone wants instant results and gratification, but when it comes to breaking your sugar addiction, you need to play the long game. What does that mean? It means adjusting your expectations such that you don't *need* to see immediate results. If you're in this for the long haul, meaning that the changes you're making are long-term changes in your behaviors regarding food, and how you think about the foods you put in your body, then what happens in the aggregate, over time, is what matters. For changes to happen long-term, they take time. Just like it took time to develop bad habits around sugar (like using it to self-soothe), it takes time to make healthier habits. Be patient with yourself!

Rule 2: A Slipup Is Not Your Excuse to Give Up

No quitters. No starting over tomorrow. Or next week. If you find that you maybe ate something you realize later you didn't want to, or that you had a misstep and dove into a pint of ice cream because you got stressed out at work or home, or because of a crisis (big or small), that doesn't mean you ditch your efforts. All too often, when we have a slipup or setback we use it as an excuse to throw in the towel. No more! I am going to help you to see how slipups are a learning tool. By identifying the *why* behind a poor food choice, you are going to be able to use this to your advantage and be better equipped for when you encounter a similar situation in the future. Trust me, the best learning comes from learning from our mistakes.

Rule 3: These Steps Aren't Linear

For some reason, humans tend to view everything in life as a linear process. Think about it: "climbing the ladder," "making headway," "achieving a breakthrough." Progress and success are often viewed in this linear manner, but that isn't accurate. Life is full of setbacks and sidetracks, and those who are most successful (and happy) are the ones who are best able to cope with inevitable derailments and continue moving forward. Part of that process may involve taking a step backward, and that is okay! Wouldn't you rather take a small temporary step down off the ladder of success to regroup, as opposed to falling off the ladder altogether and having to start over? I know I would. Or to think about it another way: If you were running a marathon and noticed at mile 5 that your shoelaces were untied, would you stop and tie them so you can go on with the race safely, or would you continue and run the risk of falling and hurting yourself and having to drop out of the race?

For many people, adopting the mindset that it's okay not to fast-track yourself to succeeding with your diet goals can be a challenge. People tend to view pauses or revisiting previous steps as failures, but they are not! If you find that you're struggling with where you are, and you recognize that and can take steps to mitigate the damage by pivoting your course, then you are succeeding. I'll give more examples of this as we move through the steps, but for now, view this as a game of chess, where you may need to detour your moves at times, but that is part of the strategy of the game!

Seven Simple Steps

One major reason why so many healthy eating plans or diets don't work is because they are overwhelming. They often spell out exactly *what* to do, but not *how* to do it. That leaves you feeling overwhelmed and lost. So here we are going to work through the process of revamping your eating habits through a series of attainable—and realistic—steps, so you won't feel like you're taking on too much.

Step 1: Admit You're Addicted

At this point, you may be flirting with the idea that your compulsions, cravings, and past failures with controlling your diet *aren't* due to your lack of willpower, or your inability to get control. You may now be starting to realize that your behavior and habits around food may indicate that you have a problem with or reliance on sugar. But are you ready to admit that it might be the *A* word?

The first step to achieve your freedom from sugar is to admit that you are addicted to it. This step might be easy for some, having known that they were addicted to it for a long time. Or maybe now they realize that they have been addicted to sugar for a while, but perhaps not exactly using those words to characterize their relationship. It also might be easier for some now that you have read the first few chapters of this book and are more familiar with addiction, and the research that's been conducted that shows that sugar addiction is real. Or maybe you're still in complete denial about your addiction to sugar, and need some cold, hard data to convince you.

Either way, take the quiz (see p. 280). See your score. Odds are, you have some degree of addiction to sugar. And on the off chance that you don't meet the criteria for addiction according to this quiz, you still can be at risk. We are all at risk. Remember, we were born to be drawn to sugar, and our modern food supply and food environment has turned what was at one time a safe survival instinct into something that is slowly killing us if we don't regain control of it.

Duration: This step of taking the quiz will take you about ten minutes to accomplish, if that. But, for some people, the idea of being "addicted" to sugar can be a hard pill to swallow and might take some time to process. For so long, our society has stigmatized addiction. We now have begun to turn a corner, and most people (but not all) realize that addiction is not a moral failing, but a biological condition that results in changes in our brain and promotes addictive behaviors. Plus, for so long addiction was only associated with things like drugs and alcohol and gambling, but as you may recall from chapter 3, there's a lot of evidence now that supports that we can also be addicted to sugar in a similar manner.

After you take the quiz, I want you to sit with the results for a bit, and really think about them. Think about the questions in the quiz, and how they relate to your present diet and relationship with food. I encourage you to mull over this for a few days and consider what it means to think about sugar as an addictive substance that is harming you. You have committed to making changes that aren't necessarily going to be easy. But if you develop the right mindset and use the tools I am going to teach you, you will be successful.

Step 2: Take Stock of Your Sugar Intake

The next step in breaking free from your sugar addiction is to figure out where all of the sugar is coming from. As discussed in chapter 2, this part can be tricky, for several reasons: Sugar is hiding in plain sight. It is not always clearly disclosed on the Nutrition Facts label, and is often added to foods that are marketed as healthy. It also finds its way into foods where it has no business being: who on Earth would expect to find added sugar in a plain English muffin?

With the information you learned in chapter 2, you can now look at the foods you are eating and see which of them are contributing to your sugar addiction. Besides the obvious sweet treats, sugar can be a sneaky additive used in many foods as a preservative. Sugar often makes food more shelf-stable and manufacturers like using it because it's cheap. Don't be fooled by added sugars; even when used as a preservative, they are still sugars. A great example of this is condiments. Many condiments—including ketchup, mayo, and salad dressings—may not taste sweet, but are packed with sugar (don't worry, you don't have to ditch these—see the recipes I've created for you on pp. 250–254 for some sugar-less options for your favorite condiments). In moderation according to the serving size, they provide little sugar to our bodies, but realistically no one just has exactly two tablespoons of ketchup with a meal, and therefore it can become an important factor when breaking a sugar addiction.

Added sugar can easily be found on all ingredient labels. But don't forget that it isn't just the added sugars that are contributing to your addiction, it's the alternative sweeteners, too. So keep those in mind when you're going through this step. If you need a refresher on what these are, flip back to chapter 2.

Take stock of your food supply. First, you need to do a complete audit of the food you have at home. Go through your refrigerator and make note of all the items you have on hand. (This is also a great opportunity to give your fridge a good deep clean and toss out whatever mystery is in the Tupperware® in the back from weeks ago.) Empty the entire contents of your fridge and clean the inside. Toss anything that is expired, or that you no longer want to keep. Then take a look at what you have. Write down every item (brands, too) and record how much added sugar is in each and whether it contains an alternative sweetener. I've created a handy worksheet in the Appendix that you can use to keep track of this information (see pp. 274–275). Note that you don't need to toss the items with added sugar or alternative sweeteners in them just yet . . . that will come later. Then, put everything back in your refrigerator.

Next, do the same thing with your pantry/dry goods.

After you complete that task, sit down and take a look at which items have added sugar. We are going to highlight those, and later you'll replace them with no-added-sugar alternatives.

Three-day food diary. This exercise is done to show you where the sugar is in your diet. You can use the template that I created for you in the Appendix (pp. 276–278), or any of your favorite food tracking apps. Just make sure that the app allows you to see how much added sugar the food has. Not many apps (that I am aware of) have the capability to track all sweeteners, so you may need to make note of this part on your own.

Be brutally honest here. Try to pick the foods that you would eat in a given day; don't select healthier options just because you are tracking them. The point of this exercise is to assess what you typically eat and how much sugar you are used to eating. That way, we can make adjustments in future steps to help minimize your sugar intake, without compromising the types of foods that you like to eat.

Eating out. Most people have their go-to places that they frequent, or the typical thing that they pick off the menu if they go out to eat. People also vary in how often they dine out or order takeout. Take stock of this (see the form you can use to record this in the Appendix, p. 279). It won't be as easy to figure out how much added sugar is in foods you don't prepare yourself, but take a look at the following pages for some guidelines to consider based on the cuisine.

DINING OUT? WATCH OUT!

Sugar may be hiding in some of your most beloved takeout options.

Pizza: Even the mom-and-pop places can hide sugar in their dough and sauce! As an alternative, find a restaurant that makes pizza with cauliflower crust topped with olive oil, veggies, and a sprinkle of mozzarella cheese. If you're ordering with a group, you can cut back on added sugar by opting for white pizza, which has no tomato sauce.

Sushi: It's common for sushi restaurants to have added sugars in their sauces and rice. Eat your sushi with wasabi or ginger and plain soy sauce, instead of dipped in a sauce, and avoid any rolls that have specialty sauces inside of them. For example, eel sauce (also known as kabayaki sauce, nitsume, or unagi sauce) is a combination of sake, mirin, sugar, and soy sauce. You can also try riceless rolls—most sushi restaurants will have a few options. Or ask for your favorite roll without the rice.

Italian restaurants: Just as with pizza, sugar can hide in many of the sauces at Italian restaurants, such as marinara sauce, Alfredo sauce, and vodka sauce. Ask the server if there is sugar in the sauce before ordering. A great alternative is to go with a side of bruschetta that you can mix into your dish!

Burger joints: Although your favorite juicy burger might not have added sugar within the meat, the bun is likely packed with sugar. Luckily, this is an easy fix. Ditch the bun and ask for leaf lettuce to wrap your burger in. Also, watch out for barbecue sauce and ketchup. Instead, load your burger with more vegetables or even avocado!

Smoothie bowls: Smoothie bowls and acai bowls certainly have a percentage of sugars that are naturally occurring from fruit, but oftentimes *more* sugar gets added. Smoothie bowls can come topped with sugar-rich agave, chocolate, hazelnut spread, peanut butter, and granola. When ordering a smoothie bowl, consider toppings such as almonds, chia seeds, fresh fruit, and walnuts.

Diner breakfasts: This one may not come as a surprise, but it's certainly worth mentioning. Restaurants that serve breakfast often have a large menu full of pancakes, waffles, French toast, pastries, cinnamon rolls, muffins, and bread products—all packed with sugar. When ordering breakfast at a restaurant, it's best to stick to eggs and fresh fruit (avocado and berries are a great combo to satisfy you).

Duration: The process of taking stock of your sugar situation could take a few days. I recommend you go slow and take the time to record everything so that you can really get a sense of what you're eating, and which foods in your diet are the largest source of sugar. With this information you can then begin to remove foods and replace them with healthier alternatives. Also, I guarantee you'll be surprised more than once about a food that you've been regularly eating that has hidden sugars or sweeteners in it!

Step 3: Identify Your Triggers

Triggers can be tricky because they can come in many forms. We all have them—those little things (or maybe big) in life that happen and can send us right into the pantry to grab a few cookies. And it isn't only situations (or people) that can trigger us; sometimes, it's certain foods—those foods that once you start eating, you can't stop. These trigger foods can lead to a downward spiral of overeating. This is nothing to feel bad about; often, these foods are specifically designed by the manufacturer to be overeaten (flip back to chapter 2 for more on how processed foods are made to be extra tasty)! Trigger foods are often highly palatable, containing plenty of sugar and fat. These foods can be anything from ice cream to cookies to crackers and vary based on an individual's taste preferences.

One of the tricks about triggers is that they can more easily affect us when we are feeling low. This is important to be aware of, especially when you are in the beginning of your journey to become sugarless and may experience withdrawal symptoms (don't worry, I'll talk more about these in the next chapter and how to cope with them). But for now, be mindful that when you're in a bad mood, feeling low, or coping with the uncomfortable period of time when you may be experiencing withdrawal, don't let triggers get their way.

The thing about triggers is that they aren't always bad. Meaning that sometimes we are triggered to eat foods that aren't good for us by *good* things that happen in our life. We often use food not only to soothe ourselves when something doesn't go as planned, but also to celebrate our successes.

Let's look at some of the common triggers that people encounter that can lead to eating. I'll cover this in greater detail in chapters 5 and 6, and help you develop a plan to cope with these triggers, but the purpose here is to get you thinking about specific times (or even specific people) that lead you down a path of sugar-seeking.

Stress. Everyone experiences some level of stress in their everyday life, and this isn't always a bad thing. A moderate amount of stress can be motivating and productive. It isn't always a great idea to sit back on your heels and be complacent in life—stress activates the nervous system in a way that makes us take action, and this can be channeled into positive behaviors. For example, if your bedroom closet is in complete disarray, and you're stressed every time you try to find a particular shirt or belt because you can't easily locate it, this stress could motivate you to cope with your stressor by taking a few hours to organize your closet.

But more often in life we don't easily turn lemons into lemonade. Often, our stressors are what weigh us down and wear on us day in and day out. It doesn't always feel so great to realize a dreaded deadline is coming up faster than expected, or to know that our new boss doesn't particularly like us, and our job may be in jeopardy as a result. To cope with the unpleasant feelings of stress, people often innocently turn to food, many times choosing sweet junk foods, to distract ourselves from the situation at hand. This may seem like a harmless coping mechanism (hey, it's better than punching the wall, or downing two shots of vodka in the middle of the day, right?), but mindless munching can leave you feeling sick to your stomach and more stressed than before.

Every day we navigate through a sea of stressors. What separates people who are calm, cool, and collected from those who are frazzled and have difficulty coping with their stressors is how we appraise those stressors. In chapter 6, I'll review how to properly evaluate your stressors so that you can then appropriately react to them, so stay tuned! But your goal for now is to think about the times when you have suddenly had a sugar craving or felt the urge to dive into a dessert. Make a list of the situations where you find that you quickly turn to food, and think about whether this may be your way of coping; then answer these questions:

What happened leading up to this?

Did you have an uncomfortable interaction with someone?

Did you find yourself in a situation where you felt disorganized or not in full control?

Once you identify these situations, you can be aware of them so that when they arise again, you'll have the tools to properly appraise the situation and cope appropriately.

Reward. You deserve to celebrate your accomplishments. Acknowledging the things that you do well, especially when they are particularly challenging, is a healthy and positive habit that will improve your overall quality of life. However, associating a job well done with a cheat day treat can be a slippery slope. This is not to say that you shouldn't celebrate a graduation or promotion with a delicious dinner out; it is simply important to be aware of the addictive qualities that certain foods have and how they can hot-wire your brain to get an extreme rush, similar to many drugs. When treats and junk food become too strongly associated with reward, we can become fixated on them, and feel guilty when we eat them without deserving them. This can easily become a toxic cycle. And it can be very easy to go from rewarding yourself with an extra slice of cake for getting that promotion to suddenly rewarding yourself with that cake for just getting through the day without snapping at someone.

If you find that you've been using the reward excuse to allow yourself to eat things you've been trying to avoid, note that you are at risk for having one of your triggers become celebrating with food. So, what are you supposed to do about it? The hard truth is: stop. Food is meant to fuel and nourish our bodies, and we shouldn't give it a place of value alongside other things we accomplish in life. You have been cheating yourself by justifying your maladaptive eating behavior under the guise that you're simply being a cheerleader for yourself. Come up with other things you can use or do to reward yourself when you have done something well. Buy yourself something. Go see a show or concert. Go to the beach. Whatever you do, you need to break the association between "good job" and eating.

If you find that this habit of rewarding yourself with food is pretty ingrained, it may be because the association started when you were a child. Rewarding children with food has been commonplace for generations (believe it or not, some pediatricians *still* give out lollipops at the end of a checkup). In fact, much of what we know about the dangers of using food as a reward comes from studies of children. One study found that maternal use of food as a reward for behavior was the only feeding practice significantly associated with children's eating in the absence of hunger— meaning that when kids are given food as a reward, they are more likely to eat for reasons *other* than being hungry. These results are further supported by a study that found that children consumed more daily fat, carbohydrates, and total calories when parents used food to reward behavior than did children whose parents did not use food as a reward.

There have also been some interesting historical studies conducted that suggest that using food as a reward can be detrimental to our overall performance. In 1950, a famous researcher named Harry Harlow observed that when food rewards were introduced to monkeys completing a puzzle task, their performance went down and errors increased. In a follow-up study, food-rewarded monkeys also showed decreased interest in the puzzle task when food was removed as a reinforcer, suggesting focus moved from the activity to the reinforcer. Bottom line: when food is the reward, our intrinsic (internal) motivation becomes diminished, and we experience a decrease in enjoyment of the rewarded task. The reward is no longer in the act of our task, but rather in getting the sugar fix, and this reduces our productivity, focus, and motivation.

Routine. Our schedules and daily habits keep us on track and help us get done what needs to be done, but routines, as valuable as they are, can include bad habits as well. For example, maybe a new bakery opened across the street from your office. You stop in once to try out one of their cupcakes and soon you're a regular for your post-work pick-me-up. This habit has become part of your routine, actually changing your brain chemistry so that you are used to this action and the subsequent pleasurable response that it causes. This is where routines can go wrong and may need re-evaluation because, unfortunately, the inclusion of a sugary treat in your routine can lead you down the path of sugar dependency.

PROFESSIONAL ORGANIZATION POSITION STATEMENTS ON THE USE OF FOOD AS A REWARD FOR CHILDREN

It isn't just the research studies telling us not to use food as a reward—major professional medical organizations advise against using food as a reward, especially in children.

Organization	Position on Food as a Reward
American Academy of Pediatrics	Food should not be used as a reward or punishment. In the long term, food rewards can create more problems.
American Academy of Family Physicians	Do not provide food for comfort or as a reward.
Academy of Nutrition and Dietetics	Do not use food as a reward. Doing so sends the message that these foods are better or more valuable than healthier foods.
American Academy of Child and Adolescent Psychiatry	Do not use food as a reward.
American Psychological Association	Avoid using food as a reward for good behavior.
Mayo Clinic	As a general rule, don't use food as a reward or punishment.
Cleveland Clinic	Do not use food as a reward.
National Institutes of Health	Food as a reward is detrimental to children's health, learning, and behavior.

Sometimes, sugar in our routines is obvious (as in the bakery example above). Other times, it sneaks in right under our nose. Do you wind down in the evening by watching television and suddenly find yourself snacking on sweets? Does the routine of running kids to after-school activities while trying to manage making dinner often-times lead to eating sugar-rich foods instead of healthier ones? Think about your daily routine and the ways in which sugar has wormed its way in. Once you recognize the pattern, you can take the necessary steps to replace it with something healthier.

Duration: This is one of the steps in the journey toward sugar freedom that you will likely have to revisit. As life goes on, our situations change in ways that can add additional stressors, opportunity for rewards, or new routines in our life that cause additional triggers to arise. The key to not letting triggers get the best of you is to know how to face them head on. If you know something is going to be a trigger for you, you need to have a game plan on how you will cope with that situation when you face it. We'll revisit some more ways in which you can cope with triggers in your diet in chapter 5. But for now, be mindful of the main ones for you, so that when you encounter these foods or situations, you can pause to reflect and remind yourself that triggers can be powerful forces driving you to overeat.

Step 4: Begin with Your Beverages

Drinks can be dangerous. I'm not just talking about drinking too much alcohol and getting a little tipsy (or worse, getting a lot tipsy and causing harm to yourself or others). I am talking about *all* the beverages you consume. Many of them are bad for your health. Let's take a closer look as to why.

Drinking sugar-filled beverages is the easiest way to add unnecessary calories to your diet and tack on unwanted weight. While a daily sugary drink might seem harmless, over time these calories add up and contribute to weight gain. Why does this happen? It has to do with how the physical form of food (liquid versus solid) can impact whether you feel full.

Before we get into why liquids *don't* make you feel full, let's first take a step back and talk about what happens in your body when you start to feel full. Picture yourself eating your favorite meal. In the beginning, you're hungry, so you eat a lot. You don't have any feelings of fullness or satiety, so you continue to eat. As you eat, your stomach releases less and less of the hunger hormone known as ghrelin, so you gradually begin to feel full, slowing how much you eat until you are finally satisfied. The feeling that causes you to push your plate away and stop eating is called satiety.

The problem is that liquids don't act in the same way as solid foods do. Drinks can not only be rich in calories (which can lead to weight gain if not burned off), they also don't provide the same feeling of satisfaction compared to solid food. Therefore, replacing a 200-calorie snack with a 200-calorie drink won't make you feel full.

Overall, solid foods produce more satiety than drinks do, even if they have the same calories. Foods require chewing, which slows the rate of consumption and increases the oral sensation of the food. The increased oral sensation can enhance satiety signals. This has been observed in studies that compared how much people eat during a meal if they are given a drink (apple juice), a semi-solid (yogurt), or solid food (bread) with the same calories before the meal. When people drank their calories, they ate more during the meal. If the people ate solid food before the meal, they ate less. Therefore, liquid calories have weaker effects on satiety, which may lead to excessive calorie intake and weight gain.

Liquid calories producing less satiety and leading to excessive caloric intake is supported through population studies. From 1966 to 2005, a study found a positive association between the intake of sugar-sweetened beverages and weight gain in children and adults. Therefore, the findings indicate those who consume more sugar-sweetened beverages are more likely to gain weight.

The weight gain is because people don't compensate for the calories they drank in what they eat. For example, if one drinks 200 calories before their meal, they must eat 200 fewer calories to consume the same number of calories and maintain their weight. However, studies have shown that people don't compensate for the calories they drank in their other snacks and meals. Instead, they still eat and drink the same calories they would have if they hadn't drunk the caloric beverage beforehand. Therefore, the caloric beverage leads to an excessive calorie intake, which causes weight gain.

Bottom line: Not only are many beverages rich in calories, but they also don't provide the same feeling of fullness that food provides. Therefore, consuming your calories in the form of liquids will leave you hungrier than if you ate the same number of calories in foods. Further, because liquid calories don't fill you up the same way, you are more likely to overeat, leading to excessive calorie consumption and weight gain.

The fact that liquid calories produce less satiety than solid calories is just half of the story. There is something that can fuel you to drink more liquid calories beyond the fact that they don't make you feel full; as you have learned from the previous chapters in this book, one thing that can override your satiety without fail is sugar. And not only that, but sugar can cause us to continue to drink more and more, just because it tastes good and we are hooked on those pleasurable feelings.

Sugar also contributes to turning "good" drinks into bad ones. Let me explain. I am a big proponent of *functional beverages*. These are beverages that are sort of like multitasking in that they allow you to get multiple health benefits at the same time. For example, coffee can be a great functional beverage naturally because it contains water, and also vitamin B6, magnesium, and several antioxidants, as well as caffeine, which can help you to focus and stay alert. The problem sets in when we *dysfunction* our functional beverages. If you have a cup of coffee, and add creamer, sugar, whipped cream, and several pumps of caramel or mocha to it, you've taken away the *functional* part of your beverage and instead created something that is completely different. Don't *dysfunction* your beverages!

What do you typically drink? Water (seltzer counts) is ideal. Water has 0 calories, 0 sugar/sweetener, and is 100 percent hydrating. Our bodies are mostly water (60 percent), and we don't typically replenish enough of what we use. Drinking more water can improve your focus and clarity, and even help you to feel fuller for longer.

But it might not be so easy for you to just give up all liquids for water. And that is okay!

You may be coming into this with a history of drinking a lot of sugary drinks. Maybe your morning coffee has a few (or more) sugars in it, or you're adding flavored creamer (which is high in added sugar). Perhaps you have a soda habit and enjoy a few cans every day. Or maybe you like sweetened tea, or juices, or energy drinks. Whatever it is, it's time to take stock of what you're drinking and make some changes, as liquid sugar is the worst kind of sugar for your diet, but the easiest to identify and replace.

In the United States, sugar-sweetened beverages are the largest contributor to excess calories and added sugars. It used to be the case that sugar-sweetened beverages came in the form of soft drinks and juices, but not anymore. Nowadays, we are finding sugar in most of our beverages, including coffees, teas, energy drinks, smoothies, and yes, even water! Let's look at the different categories of beverages people typically drink and discuss some ways you can "edit" those beverages that you enjoy to make them sugarless.

Coffee

Coffee can go from a functional beverage to a full-blown sugar-bomb of a dessert in the blink of an eye. It can be a significant source of liquid calories as sugar, milk, and sweeteners are added to enhance its flavor. For example, a venti Starbucks® Iced Caffè Mocha starts at 450 calories and 43 g of sugar, and a large Dunkin'® Iced Signature Latte has 530 calories and 51 g of sugar. Yikes!

Your best bet when it comes to coffee is to have it black or with some milk. However, be mindful of your milk (plant-based milks in particular often contain added sugar—most oat or soy milks in coffee shops have added sugar in them, so be sure to inquire). If you're in the habit of adding sugar to your coffee, try cutting it out, or if that won't work for you, start cutting back on how much you add. Give it a few days and I bet you won't miss it.

Soft Drinks and Sodas

The beverage industry is booming, and when it comes to soft drinks we have lots of options these days. Many have added sugars and sweeteners, as well as caffeine. It's important to identify *why* you like a particular soft drink. Is it the caffeine? Try coffee instead (see above). Is it the bubbles? Then maybe give seltzer a try (many different flavors are available). Or try sparkling water or mineral water. If you're drinking soda because you like the liquid sugar, you just need to stop because this is probably the worst thing you can be doing to yourself when it comes to trying to break up with sugar.

Popular soft drinks in the United States are loaded with calories and sugar (and not much else in terms of nutrients). For example, a 20-oz serving of Mountain Dew® has 77 g of sugar, a 16-oz peach Snapple® bottle has 40 g of sugar, and 12 oz of ginger ale (known for its so-called benefits for when you're under the weather) contains 34 g of sugar. Soft drinks are also known to disguise their added sugars as other names in their ingredients list, including high-fructose corn syrup, dextrose, and maltose. This not only makes it even harder to detect sugars in drinks unless you're a seasoned label reader, but it also means there are harmful processing methods and chemicals used to produce these products.

Energy Drinks

The most common reason why people drink energy drinks is for, well, energy, of course. These beverages often contain more caffeine than coffee (dangerously more in some cases), along with other vitamins and ingredients that can be healthy. However, they all contain sweeteners of some sort—you need sugar or a sweetener to mask the awful taste of the added caffeine and B vitamins. So what can you do if you're hooked on these drinks? I suggest switching to coffee or tea, which contain a more reasonable amount of caffeine, and you can control what you add to it. Energy drinks are typically

WATCH OUT FOR THAT VALUE MEAL!

If you value your health, you'll skip the value meal. Fast-food restaurants often include drinks in their combo value meals to entice people to buy them because they are getting "a deal." A study found that the default drinks included in a combo meal at McDonald's® averaged about 52 g of sugar, 48 g at Burger King®, and 35 g at Wendy's®. Alone, a McDonald's® small vanilla milkshake racks up about 480 calories and 51 g of sugar, so these averages are only the beginning of sugary items on common fast-food menus. These sugary calories are being added to what is already a high-calorie, high-fat meal. The additional calories that come from these beverages accumulate into a surplus of calories consumed.

consumed cold or at room temperature, so if you aren't a hot coffee fan, try iced coffee.

Here are a few examples of energy drinks that are loaded with added sugar. Any benefit you think you are getting from the *energy* in them will quickly be reversed by the *energy drain* from the sugar crash you'll experience soon after drinking one of these, so think twice! For example, a 16-oz Monster Energy® Drink has 200 calories and 27 g of sugar, Red Bull® Energy Drink has 212 calories and 50 g of sugar, and Rockstar Energy® Drink has 280 calories and 63 g of sugar. Looking back at the Rockstar Energy® example, 63 g of sugar equates to 15 tsps of sugar. That's about how much sugar is found in six Krispy Kreme® Original Glazed Doughnuts or twelve Oreo® cookies!

Juices

Juice is often seen as a children's drink, but it is not recommended for kids—or adults! In fact, the American Academy of Pediatrics (AAP) has changed its stance on juice and now recommends that infants and toddlers not be given any juice, and even older kids should have a very limited amount, if any at all. The reason is because juice is highly processed and the fruit itself is stripped of nearly all its nutritional benefits. There is no longer fiber, and therefore it requires little to no mechanical digestion from the mouth (chewing). This makes it yet another high source of liquid sugar in our diets, and one that is easy to overconsume.

Juice can be very deceiving because often it is sweetened naturally with the sugar that it contains, not *added* sugar. However, juice should still be avoided because it is basically just a concentrated form of sugar. For example, if you were to drink a 10-oz glass of apple juice, that would be the equivalent of two apples. But you aren't getting the nutritional benefits of those apples—just the sugar! Some other popular juices that might seem healthy but are loaded with sugar are Tropicana® orange juice, which is 110 calories and contains 22 g of sugar per 8 fl oz; Welch's® grape juice, at 140 calories and 36 g of sugar per 8 fl oz; and Ocean Spray® cranberry juice, with 100 calories and 23 g of sugar per 8 fl oz.

If you are a juice drinker, and you don't think you can give it up easily, I suggest you start off by diluting it with water or seltzer. It might taste less sweet at first, but after a few days your taste buds will get used to it and you won't even miss the sweeter stuff. Another option is to forget the juice, and switch to a smoothie. You get much more nutrition from the *whole* fruit, as opposed to just the juice.

Smoothies

Smoothies are a great way to get veggies and fruits into your diet and better than juices because you're retaining the fiber and other nutrients that are typically tossed out when juicing. However, be aware that you often can be gulping down a lot more fruit than you would ever be able to eat in one sitting. For example, a Naked® Strawberry Banana Smoothie contains juice from 22 strawberries, 1¾ apples, 1⅓ bananas, and a hint of orange. So, drink your smoothie slowly!

Like other beverages, liquid foods go down much faster and easier than solid foods, so you may not feel full after having a smoothie as a meal. If that's the case, try changing things up and instead of making a smoothie, make yourself a fruit and veggie salad using the ingredients that you would typically blend up. It is a completely different experience!

One thing to remember when you are choosing lower-sugar options in your diet is that premade smoothies are *not* the same as a homemade smoothie. At home, you can ensure that there are no sweeteners added to your smoothies (aside from the naturally occurring sweetness of the whole fruit), and you can play around with the ingredients to make it healthy and satisfying. Try using different types of milks, unsweetened nut milk alternatives, or yogurt. Use whole fresh fruit or frozen, along with fresh or frozen veggies like zucchini, spinach, or kale. I always recommend adding some veggies to your smoothie—even if you aren't a veggie fan, you won't even taste them! Also, to get even more out of your smoothie, try adding a tablespoon of all-natural nut butter for healthy fats.

But when you're purchasing a smoothie, be on the lookout for added sugars. For example, the Pure Recharge Strawberry smoothie from Smoothie King® contains 26 g of added sugar, a Mango Magic smoothie from Tropical Smoothie Cafe® contains 44 g of added sugar, and a strawberry parfait smoothie from Bolthouse Farms® contains 29 g of added sugar.

Drinkable Yogurts

Drinkable yogurts are advertised mostly for children but have begun to make their way into an on-the-go alternative for adults as well. And, as you probably guessed, the main issue with drinkable yogurts is that they contain added sugar. Added sugar in yogurt can turn a healthy snack into a full-on dessert and can be especially dangerous. For example, one Chobani® drinkable yogurt contains 7 g of added sugar, with few other nutritional components.

This doesn't mean you have to knock all yogurts off your radar. Yogurt can be a great high-protein snack with added probiotics to benefit your gut health. But stop drinking your yogurt—the sugarless options are not typically drinkable. Instead, look for plain yogurts with no added sugar, and you can make your own "drinkable" version if you like by combining some fruit, yogurt, and a splash of milk in a blender.

Milks

It used to be that the only kind of milk you would see in the grocery store was cow's milk, but that has changed! There is now a large variety to choose from when picking a milk—everything from oat milk to macadamia nut milk to hemp milk. What do you need to keep in mind about all of these milks if you are being mindful of your added sugar intake?

Dairy milk does in fact contain sugar—naturally occurring sugar called lactose. Metabolically, our bodies digest lactose differently from glucose. Lactose is broken down by an enzyme called lactase that is created by our bodies essentially to digest breast milk as a newborn. As we age, our bodies make less lactase, and therefore many people become lactose sensitive or even lactose intolerant in some cases. Although lactose differs from

BUT I'M VEGAN. HOW CAN I BEAT MY SUGAR ADDICTION WITHOUT ALL THE CARBS?

A vegan diet usually includes carbohydrate-rich foods—and it should—because a vegan is cutting out a large portion of other foods. Although it can be more carb-focused, it doesn't have to be filled with sugar-rich and processed foods! There are an abundance of whole-food sources of proteins, fats, and carbs for vegans while managing a sugar addiction. Great sources of protein to include in a whole food–based vegan diet are tofu, tempeh, and legumes. Increasing your plant-based protein will allow you to overcome sugar cravings more effectively than filling your plate with starchy carbs. Carbs like whole grains (quinoa, brown rice, farro, bulghur), fruits, and vegetables will give your body essential micronutrients and fiber to promote optimal health, digestion, and satiation. Including high-protein and high-fiber foods in your vegan lifestyle will allow your brain to forget it even wants sugar.

other forms of sugars, I put this type of sugar into the category of naturally occurring sugars in fruit. Yes, it still impacts our blood sugar, but with less effect due to the combination of protein and

WHICH ALCOHOLIC BEVERAGES ARE BEST WHEN CUTTING SUGAR?

Alcoholic beverages can be a sneaky source of added sugar. Mixed drinks are often the culprits, with a 4-oz margarita having an average of 168 calories and 28 g of sugar, 7 oz of piña colada having 536 calories and 43 g of sugar, and 6 oz of mojito having 143 calories and 26 g of sugar.

If you still want to enjoy an occasional alcoholic beverage, without all the sugar, there are many alternatives. Some vodka sodas are made with real fruit juice (not ideal, but the amount of sugar in the juice is much less than what you would find in most mixed drinks) and no artificial sweeteners. Craving a margarita? An alternative to a traditional margarita is to use one serving of mezcal tequila, fresh lime juice, and soda water. It's refreshing, without the added sugar from a premade mix or simple syrup!

Hard alcohols like tequila, gin, whiskey, and brandy are also good options if you want to sip on them. However, most people enjoy these with a mixer (which is where all the sugar hides), so think about making your own drink with ice, soda water, and a splash of one of these—you can also add fresh lime juice.

fat that comes along with milk. So, unless you are lactose sensitive or intolerant, there isn't a sugar-based reason why you need to avoid drinking dairy milks. But be aware that flavored dairy milks, like chocolate or strawberry milk, do contain added sugars, so skip those!

It's a bit easier to spot added sugar in plant-based milk alternatives. These milks are made with water and blended with a nut, seed, or legume. Many popular nut milk brands add sugar, brown rice syrup, or other forms of sweeteners to their milks to make them more palatable. For example, Almond Breeze® vanilla almond milk contains 13 g of sugar per cup. When purchasing a plant-based milk, it's important to look for the unsweetened variety, to avoid unwanted added sugars in your diet. Plus, you'll be surprised to find the sugar-free ones don't taste all that different—especially if you're using them as a milk substitute in coffee or with your morning cereal or smoothie.

So, How Do You Get Started with Revamping Your Beverages?

The first step is to start with your food diary and see which beverages you're consuming. Make a list where you order them based on added sugar. Let's start there.

First thing I want you to do is really think about that drink, and why you like it. Is it the bubbles? The buzz? Or the sweet taste? There are a variety of reasons why we like certain beverages. Each of

WHAT ABOUT WINE?

Naturally occurring sugars in wine come from the grapes used to create the wine itself. These grapes are fermented until the sugar turns into alcohol and eventually a distinct flavor that we know as wine! However, many wines nowadays contain added sugars for flavor and are not aged as long as quality wines we typically see in Europe and the Mediterranean.

What can you drink if you like wine? Instead of pouring a glass of American-made Moscato, try a dry red variety or a dry white. These wines contain the least amount of residual sugar and usually have less added sugar, if any. There are also brands like FitVine® that make wine varieties with less than 1 g of sugar per serving.

these reasons is important to understand, as they can help us revise our drinks to make them better for us.

Maybe the reason you like a particular beverage has nothing to do with the taste (at first blush), but rather, you like it because of how it makes you feel. Coffee is a great example here—it is naturally bitter, and therefore typically aversive in terms of taste. I remember being a kid and my mom letting me taste her coffee for the very first time. It was gross! I wondered, *How can she drink this stuff?* As I have learned later in life as a coffee drinker myself, she didn't necessarily drink the coffee for the taste (at first), she drank it because she liked how it made her feel. She came to like the taste of coffee not because of the actual taste, but because of the association it had with giving her a little pep and energy. If I were to play a trick on her and secretly swap out her regular coffee for decaf for a few days, odds are she would start to like the taste less and less, because it wouldn't have the same impact on how it made her feel.

So, really think about why you like to drink what you drink, and how or if sugar plays a role. If your daily routine involves a can of soda at lunch and a cocktail at dinner, rework your associations to those sugary drinks away from your normal routine. This can definitely take time and effort, but rethinking your drinks will pay off for your health, longevity, and well-being! Instead, replace those drinks with ones that have no sugar and eventually, your brain won't notice the difference.

Duration: It will depend on how much sugar you're drinking. Some people move through this step fast because they aren't really drinking much sugar to begin with, while others require more time. If you're in the latter group, know that if you are incrementally cutting out sugar from your beverages, you're making big progress. Start off with the beverage you're drinking most often, and once you've successfully figured out a sugarless swap, move on to tackle the next one.

Step 5: Breaking Down Breakfast

The most important meal of the day is also the one that often contains the most sugar.

Eating a healthy breakfast will kick-start your metabolism and help burn more calories throughout the day. Although opinions on this topic vary, one factor remains steady—individuals who eat breakfast regularly consume significantly more nutrients than those who skip it. Furthermore, eating breakfast can enhance cognitive performance, which highlights how vital consuming breakfast can be for mental functioning. Eating breakfast allows us to get more nutrients and more energy, which may correspond to better health outcomes.

For these reasons, breakfast is often touted as "the most important meal of the day." However, many people skip it. Whether it's a lack of time or not feeling hungry first thing in the morning, many people bypass breakfast and go straight to lunch. However, this is not a good idea for a few reasons. First, research shows that people who don't eat breakfast oftentimes miss out on key micronutrients like vitamin D and calcium, as well as iron and folate. Plus, not only is eating breakfast associated with lower risk of chronic diseases, it may have a positive effect on memory and attention, too.

Although there are benefits to incorporating breakfast into your daily routine, it's also an easy way to accidentally start your day with a bowlful of sugar. That might be why breakfast isn't always recommended for weight loss purposes. In fact, some research shows that people who eat breakfast actually have a more difficult time losing weight than those who skip it. I am not at all suggesting that you forgo breakfast if you want to lose weight, but anyone who's gone this route and lost weight probably did so because they were cutting sugar out of their diet—not necessarily because they were skipping the meal.

In the US, breakfast has morphed into dessert. While some foods like cinnamon buns and doughnuts are obviously loaded with added sugar, and not typically what you would pick if you're cutting sugar out of your diet, other foods are a lot sneakier. Yogurt with granola, bran muffins, and cereals are often thought of as healthful options but can be just as high in sugar as some pastries. Plus, if your mornings are super busy, but you don't want to skip breakfast, convenience may be the top priority. The food industry knows this and is happy to "help." There are tons of prepackaged, single-serve cereals and oatmeals to pick from, as well as a vast assortment of frozen waffles and pancakes, all of which typically have added sugar.

Now let's look at some beverages many people have first thing in the morning. We covered this in Step 4, but it's worth reviewing again, as beverages are often a big part of breakfast routines. For one, if you're drinking juice, stop! Ounce for ounce, some juices, and especially juice "cocktails," have the same amount of sugar as soda. Next up is milk and milk alternatives. Some have upward of 20 g of sugar per cup. Some milk alternatives, like oat and rice milk, usually have a lot of sugar, but if your nut milk is sweetened, it can have just as much. Don't be fooled by the addition of vitamins, either. Certain milk alternatives and juices are fortified with vitamins and minerals; however, not all of them are stable and actually lose many of those nutrients during processing. Unfortunately, the nutrition label doesn't necessarily reflect the vitamin content at the time you're drinking it. Lastly, consider your coffee. If you drink it black or with a splash of milk or cream, no need to worry at all because coffee is naturally sugar-free. However, if you enjoy a flavored creamer, one tablespoon is about the same as two packs of sugar.

What can you do to revamp your breakfast? If you're thinking about your typical morning breakfast and seeing a lot of added sugar now, don't fret. While there's no denying that most breakfast foods are high in sugar, there are also plenty of healthful choices as well. But navigating the breakfast aisle can be a challenge. So what should you start your day with? In general, choose breakfast foods that are high in protein and fiber, while being low in sugar. Both protein and fiber have a satiating effect and also keep blood sugar levels from spiking. Eggs, the US's second-favorite breakfast item, are an excellent choice. They are sugar-free and are one of the only foods that naturally contain vitamin D, which is good for your bone health, brain health, and also your immune system. And don't be afraid to eat the yolk—it contains protein as well as antioxidants and fat-soluble vitamins, and we know through recent research that eggs are not a significant source of bad cholesterol. Plus, there are so many ways to prepare them. Scramble them with veggies, serve them sunny-side up, or poach them. Make a batch of hard-boiled eggs before the weekend ends as an easy breakfast for hectic weekday mornings (unpeeled, they last for seven days in the fridge. If you want to peel them in advance to save time, they last five days). If hard-boiled eggs aren't your thing, make oven-baked eggs in muffin tins. Add in whatever fixings you want—cheese, spinach, onions and mushrooms, zucchini, or bell peppers. These can also be made in advance and stored for up to four days in the fridge. Occasionally adding cheese to your eggs or omelets can promote fullness and provide the body with additional nutrients. For example, adding one slice of cheddar cheese to your scrambled eggs at breakfast can add 3.96 g of protein, 120 mg of calcium, 0.624 mg of zinc, and 13.1 mg of potassium.

If you're not an egg person, either due to an allergy or preference, there are plenty of other low-sugar breakfast choices. Greek yogurt has gained a lot of attention over the years due to its high-protein, low-sugar content. It's thick and creamy and naturally low in lactose compared to other dairy products due to the straining process (which is great for people who are lactose intolerant). One cup of plain Greek yogurt provides about 17 g of protein and only 6 g of naturally occurring sugar (lactose). Just be careful to read the label of the flavored ones because the sugar content can jump to more than 20 g due to added sugars in some cases. If you're not a fan of the tart flavor, add your own fresh fruit to give it some sweetness. Berries are one of the best choices due to their naturally high fiber content. Besides fruit, you can add a dollop of any nut butter of your choice with chia seeds or flax for a high-fiber crunch.

Speaking of fruit, one word of caution. Don't try to "save" calories by just eating fruit alone for breakfast. Not only will this cause you to be hungry right away, but it will also cause your blood sugar levels to spike and fall more than they would if you had a balanced meal. If you're going to have fruit for breakfast, be sure to pair it with some protein and fat.

Then there's always classic oatmeal. There are so many varieties it's hard to know which one is best. Instant oats are processed in such a way that our body actually digests it quicker than steel-cut oats, so if you have the time, steel-cut oats are superior to instant ones. However, if you're on a time crunch, instant oats are still a great option, providing 4 g of fiber (just make sure they're plain). Throw in some walnuts or peanut butter, banana, and cinnamon to add some healthy fat, antioxidants, and of course flavor—because plain oats are pretty bland on their own. The addition of fat and protein from the nuts will help slow digestion and help satiate you for longer compared to eating oats on their own. This can help you ward off sugar cravings, too!

Hopefully you're convinced that breakfast can be easy and healthy. These are just some ideas to get you started. Flip ahead to page 214 to see some low-to-no sugar recipes that I've developed as a perfect start for your breakfast.

INTERMITTENT FASTING: IS IT GOOD FOR BATTLING SUGAR ADDICTION?

In short, no, and for many reasons. Intermittent fasting is the act of cyclical fasting that can be done daily or weekly. This type of dietary pattern allows your body to use ketones instead of glucose as its main fuel source. It sounds good in theory but can often lead to excessive cravings and bingeing on unhealthy foods, like those with a lot of sugar. By restricting your body of calories and nutrients, your brain automatically will crave quick energy sources—like sugar! This can be especially harmful for those dealing with sugar addiction because it can throw your hormones and regulatory mood functions into a cake-and-cookies spiral. The best rule to follow instead of intermittent fasting is to eat protein-dense snacks and meals when your hunger cues call. For example, a balanced first meal of the day that includes things like eggs and avocado will do much more good to your hormones and brain than skipping breakfast altogether.

Duration: Much like the situation with beverages, how long it will take you to de-sugar your breakfast routine will depend on where you are coming into this. For many people, this step will be relatively easy because they are in the habit of drinking their breakfast (smoothies, coffee drinks, yogurt drinks, etc.), so they'll have tackled this in Step 4. But for others, it may take more time.

Remember, this isn't a race. You want to make good decisions, and choices that you can stick with moving forward. The goal isn't to deprive yourself, but rather, to slowly incorporate better options into your diet to help reduce your sugar dependence. So give this step a week or two, at minimum, and make sure that you're on track with a realistic breakfast plan before you move on to Step 6. I suggest having three to four go-to breakfast options and rotating among them. Make sure that one of them is a quick fix (a smoothie, for example, if you need to take breakfast to go), and one is friendly for when dining out (my go-to when having breakfast out is black coffee, one egg over easy, a side of fruit, and a side of bacon that I split with the table).

Step 6: De-sugar Your Dinner

Now that we have breakfast down, let's tackle dinner. It might seem like I'm skipping something here (lunch, where are you?), but I'll come back to that in Step 7. I'm jumping ahead to dinner because going in this order of attack will help to lessen any feelings of deprivation. If you focus at first on your morning and evening meals, it

WHAT'S FOR DINNER?

If you're craving a hamburger or sandwich, there are a few different options to consider. There are an abundance of low-carb wraps and breads on the market today that can provide fewer total carbohydrates than traditional breads—which typically contain added sugars in addition to other carbohydrates. Another idea is to use only half of the bun or wrap. Lettuce leaves in place of buns have also gained popularity recently, and can be a nice way to cut the amount of sugars you're consuming. If soups are a go-to of yours, don't worry. Soups can still be enjoyed; you may just need to pay closer attention to the food label. Creamy soups tend to have more added sugar in them, so watch out for those!

allows time in between for you to regroup. So here, in Step 6, I'll help you figure out how your dinner may be adding sugar to your diet, and offer ideas for swaps to your favorite dishes to make them healthier and less addicting.

Get Your Greens

Not everyone loves them, but greens are an important part of your dinner for a few reasons. First, they contain nutrients that our brains and bodies need to function and stay well. But even more important for our purposes, they will help you feel full. If you can get into the routine of incorporating greens (kale, lettuce, broccoli, spinach— literally any green veggie) into your diet, you will 1) satisfy your urge to eat something, 2) get fiber and nutrients to help you feel full, and 3) not send your blood sugar levels out of whack—since greens are very blood-sugar friendly. All this means that eating greens will help to mitigate your sugar cravings and help you to resist the urge to dig into sugar.

It is always a good idea to try to incorporate a big green salad into your day, and dinner is the perfect time to do so. The possibilities that can come from salad are endless. Salads aren't always just a pile of lettuce—you can get creative and add just about anything to your greens. When constructing your dish, start with some sort of greens as the base—your salad can consist of spinach, kale, romaine, or even a spring mix. Vegetables such as carrots, peppers, onions, and broccoli are great additions. Also, crushed-up nuts or seeds are a great way to add some protein, healthy fats, and crunch. If you have leftover cooked veggies from the previous night, add them! Who said that your salad needs to be raw, or even that it has to be cold.

I recommend starting off every dinner with a salad. No, you don't need to *only* have salad for dinner, but you should get into the habit of starting with one. But of course, you can turn your salad into a full meal by adding protein like grilled chicken, meat, fish (cold salmon is my favorite), or tofu. Additional add-ons can include quinoa, cheese, beans, and fruits. Really, the possibilities are endless! And remind yourself that salads aren't boring unless you make them that way!

Salads start to go sour when we start talking about salad dressing. Salad dressing *can* be a nice addition to your salad as long as you keep a close eye on the nutrition label. Companies will often promote salads as "fat-free," but excess sugar is added to make up for the lack of taste. Just a little olive oil, lemon juice, and salt and pepper may be all you need if you've composed a nice salad with lots of goodies already. Or think about adding a spoonful of salsa or hummus to your salad instead of dressing. Also, check out the sugarless salad dressing recipes on pages 242, 252, and 253. These are great to have on hand.

Choosing Your Entrée

The goal when choosing your dinner entrée is to opt for something with no sugar, but also to enjoy a meal that will keep you feeling full and satisfied. There are many entrée options to select from that are high in protein, low in sugar, and packed with micronutrients. Some entrée options include turkey, chicken, meatloaf, steak, fish, etc. One small grilled chicken breast, without the skin, can provide the body with roughly 31.1 g of protein, 0 g of sugar, 7.35 mg of calcium, and 10.6 mg of niacin. Pairing this chicken breast with a steamed vegetable of your choice, along with brown rice, can provide essential nutrients that the body needs. Choosing fish, like salmon, for an entrée can provide

DIPS AND SAUCES

Like salad dressings, dips and sauces can be loaded with added sugar, and they can quickly turn your well-intentioned meal into a sugar-soaked one. When eating out and ordering an entrée, ask if it's prepared in a sauce, and if so, ask for it on the side. That way, you can have some, but your meal doesn't need to take a bath in it. A good option is to ask for a side of drawn butter in lieu of whatever sauce your meal was meant to contain—that way, you can have something savory to add, but know that it doesn't contain sugar.

around 25.7 g of protein, varying amounts of omega-3 fatty acids, 461 mg of potassium, and 39.4 μg of selenium. I'm sure this isn't the first time you've heard someone suggest eating chicken and steamed veggies, and maybe that sounds super boring to you. Well, don't let it! Knowing that you are fueling your body with protein and healthy nutrients that will help you to avoid craving sugar should be exciting! Look at these foods as your tools to help you get off sugar and get on track with your health goals. Plus, you can easily turn boring chicken and vegetables into something exciting by using spices, which are a great way to customize and flavor your dinner without adding sugar. Also, you can use sugar-free condiments to jazz up just about any dish.

Duration: This step may take up to a few weeks to complete. Coming up with your own personal dinner menu is a must. Think of it like a menu you would see at a restaurant, but with items that are customized toward you and your life. You should have three to four dinner meal ideas that you can make at home, and three to four options when eating out at a restaurant. Planning is key! If you have a vague idea of what you want to make or eat for dinner, be sure you have the ingredients to prepare it. If you wait until the last minute, you end up making whatever you have on hand, and that might not be the best option for you. If you have your go-to meals in mind, make sure that you have those ingredients in the house so you can prepare them. Need some ideas? Check out the recipes on pages 216–268 and the kitchen staples list on pages 212–213 for some ideas to help you get started.

Step 7: Lunch and Snacks

Lunch is a meal that can often be interchangeable with dinner. The key to cutting back on sugar for lunch is to keep your favorite meals but modify them appropriately. For example, if one of your frequent lunch meals is a BLT on whole-wheat bread, you can alter this to contain less sugar by swapping out the bread for one with no added sugar, or reconstruct it by using a lettuce wrap on the outside and adding some sliced avocado to accompany the bacon and tomato on the inside. This way, you can still enjoy your favorite meal but in a way that contains less sugar. Let's talk about some more ways you can make sure that your lunch has less sugar and is more nutritious!

My advice for lunch is to keep it super simple. Think about your typical day and how lunch fits into it. If you work during the day and don't have much time to eat lunch (let alone prepare it), then opt for simple salads, like egg salad, tuna salad, or chicken salad. All of these options are relatively high in protein to keep you feeling full, and you can customize them to include extra things that you like to your taste. For example, I love to have canned tuna mixed with a little olive oil, capers, a splash of lemon juice, and some cracked pepper. There is zero sugar in it, and a lot of protein and healthy fats—and I can make it in a flash. Another tip—anytime we have chicken for dinner, the leftovers immediately become chicken salad for lunch the next day. Just pick apart the leftover chicken, and then add what you like. I throw in chopped celery (or celery seed if I don't have any fresh celery on hand), some mayo (make sure it's no sugar added), chopped onion, and pepper to make the base, but you can get creative and add anything from grapes to diced apples to sweeten it up.

Even something as simple as a peanut butter sandwich can still be enjoyed while cutting back on sugar. Instead of using two slices of white bread, you can use only one, or swap it with a no-added-sugar option. You also want to make sure that your peanut butter is just peanuts (check the label). Adding bananas and a sprinkle of cinnamon to your peanut butter sandwich can enhance the flavor,

DOUBLE-UP YOUR DINNER

One way to make double duty of your healthy dinner is to make more than you plan to eat so there's enough for lunch the next day. This is a great way to cut back on your work (one less meal to think about or prepare) and ensure you have something healthy ready for the next day. Get into the habit of immediately preparing your lunch for the next day when cleaning up your dinner by loading up your to-go container with the leftovers.

promote fullness, and keep you excited. Yes, adding bananas and cinnamon to a peanut butter sandwich *can* be exciting, especially when you know it will help you to break your addiction to sugar.

For many people, the trouble with eating a healthy lunch is that we 1) typically eat lunch on-the-go (i.e., quickly, while working or running errands or taking care of the kids), or 2) we dine out. When we rush through lunch and don't plan out something healthy to eat, but instead grab the closest thing to use when hunger strikes, we run the huge risk of going for sugars. This is because our brains have been trained to know that we'll get a quicker energy rush from the carbs.

When dining out, we are often faced with two hurdles. First, the food in many restaurants is generally less healthy, and you have less control over what actually ends up in your dish. Second, we tend to view dining out as "a treat" and are tempted to use this as an occasion to celebrate with food. And people can find many reasons to celebrate—anything from "we finished that project" to "it's Tuesday!" can be all the justification we need to push us away from our healthy eating goals and dive into a sugary drink or meal.

This is why you need a plan! Don't go out to lunch with your friend and have no idea what you're going to order when you get there. Pretty much every restaurant has their menus online, so check it out ahead of time and think about what you're going to order. If you frequent a coffee shop or bagel place, have your order in mind before you arrive.

Now that we've tackled lunch, let's talk about snacking. Snacks can be one of the most challenging areas of your diet to adjust when reducing sugar. TV commercials, convenience stores, supermarket checkout aisles, and vending machines all entice us to eat. Having access to a variety of snacks, both healthy and unhealthy, can make it more difficult to realize exactly what you are consuming. Although snacking can be problematic, it doesn't mean we need to omit this portion of our diet. In fact, snacks are a vital part of our day to keep us satiated and energized. The key, when snacking, is to choose foods with a high nutritional value and consume them in reasonable amounts.

A good place to start when discovering low-sugar snacks is fruits and vegetables. I know, I know . . . not what you were hoping to read. If you are coming out of your relationship with sugar, odds are you aren't going to be super happy to swap your caramel popcorn for carrots and celery sticks. But think of it this way—snacks are meant to fuel you with nutrients and calories when you need them. They aren't meant to be your source of happiness or joy. If you're eating healthy snacks, you will get true joy from how you are treating and caring for your body. And many healthy snacks *are* satisfying to eat, but we often forget this when we're comparing them to the typical junk food snacks. Remember, don't put gasoline in the Tesla!

Fruits and vegetables contain an abundance of vitamins, minerals, and fiber, and can even lower your risk of chronic diseases. Some options to consider are celery with natural peanut butter or hummus on top, a sliced apple with natural almond butter, toast or a few crackers with guacamole (avocado, onion, cilantro, lime juice, and tomatoes), yogurt bark with berries (check out the recipe on p. 257), or even a handful of nuts. Fruits and vegetables tend to be high in fiber, which is known to promote satiety. For example, one raw peach can provide 2.25 g of fiber, and one raw pear can provide 5.58 g of fiber. Fiber is your friend, and actually your *best friend* when trying to avoid sugar cravings!

As previously discussed, high-protein food options can leave us feeling fuller longer and can help maintain blood sugar levels. A great high-protein snack option is any type of nuts. Nuts are a food that you can grab whenever you're in a hurry but that are still packed with nutrients. For example, a small 100-calorie package of almonds provides 3.64 g of protein, 46.6 mg of calcium, 124 mg of potassium, and 48.4 mg of magnesium. Other high-protein snack options are sliced turkey, beef or chicken jerky, hard-boiled eggs, string cheese, or tuna.

One of the largest barriers to healthy snacking is that snacks are typically needed when we're in a rush. When we are on-the-go, prepackaged foods can seem like a reasonable solution. Snacks that are easy to grab are usually the worst for us: candy bars, potato chips, most granola bars, etc. Preparing snacks ahead of time is the easiest way to overcome this barrier. Portioning nuts, fruits, or vegetables into reclosable bags or containers is a good idea. Pop some popcorn at home and add your own toppings (like salt or Old Bay® Seasoning), then portion it out into snack bags. Having these snacks prepared ahead of time can promote their convenience and make you more inclined to choose them when in a hurry.

Protein bars, granola bars, or breakfast bars are commonly thought to be healthy snack options. They're considered to be a healthy choice because they sound healthier than grabbing cookies. But the truth is, you'd be better off eating a cookie! If you take a

MAKE NEW HEALTHY HABITS

This book is all about reframing your health habits. Part of that means developing some new habits. If the idea of having portioned-out bags of chopped fruits and veggies as snacks sounds great but just never seems to happen in your house, change that! Make it happen. Find a dedicated time every few days to chop and bag some snacks. Have a spot in your pantry for the room-temp snacks, and a spot in the fridge for the cold ones. I do this after we go grocery shopping—before I put everything away. Also, this is a great task for kids—little ones can sort snacks into bags, and your teen can chop veggies and fruit.

close look at any type of bar's food label, it tends to be high in carbohydrates and sugar, which can impede your goals. For example, one CLIF Bar® can have up to 21.5 g of sugar. With the previously mentioned options available, it is best practice to always read the food label before purchasing.

Duration: This last step may take the longest. That's because lunch and snacks are the least predictable parts of our diets, and usually the

GOODBYE, SNACK ATTACK!

You may find that once you reduce the added sugar in your diet, the urgency of your snack attacks will become less and less. This is because when you get off of the sugar roller coaster, your body won't be struggling with surges and dips in blood sugar and dopamine, which typically are what lead us to crave a snack all of a sudden.

most difficult to plan. I suggest you give this step a few weeks, and if you find that it's too much to manage your snacks *and* lunch together, focus on the snacks first.

▶•◀

There you have it! Seven simple steps to sugar freedom! Okay, maybe they aren't all that simple in practice, but in theory they are, and this is your guide. While you're working through these steps, you may find that some things hold you up or temporarily set you back. Next, we're going to discuss some of these common hurdles in depth so that you can cope with them when they arise.

CHAPTER 5

HANDLING THE HURDLES: TRIGGERS, WITHDRAWAL, AND CRAVINGS

I never said this was going to be easy. In life, is anything that is really worth it ever actually easy?

I have come to learn that something being "easy" is a hindsight observation. Think about all the things you've accomplished so far in your life, and how you felt while you were going through them. Getting through college, having a baby, a marriage, buying a house, etc. All these things are super difficult and take a lot of work, but once we're on the other side of them, we tend to view them as not being so bad after all.

You can soon add sugar addiction to this list. It isn't easy, and you'll be tempted to throw in the towel and give up, but don't, because once you're on the other side, you'll be glad that you didn't give up. The discomfort you may feel when working through these steps to break free from sugar isn't going to last forever, but I guarantee that the sense of accomplishment and joy you feel when you do break free will be something that you are extremely proud of and will carry with you.

Let's look at some of the hurdles that you can expect to encounter along the way. First off, let's talk about some of the triggers that can lead us to eating sugar.

Top Triggers

In chapter 4, I talked about how stress, reward, and routine can be common triggers for eating sugar. We'll talk in more detail about dealing with stress in the next chapter, as stress is a common reason why people overeat and often turn to sugar. Now, let's talk about what you can do to cope with other triggers if you encounter them, or what you can do to avoid them altogether. Learning to acknowledge triggers that can send us sugar-spiraling, as well as knowing how to manage and overcome their temptation, is a critical tool to use in your sugar-less journey!

Tips on Navigating Triggers

Before you can start combatting triggers, you must first assess what your personal triggers are. Do you feel at a bit of a loss right now because you don't exactly know what your personal triggers are? Don't worry, I'm here to help. Sometimes, our triggers aren't always clear, but they can become clearer when you evaluate your situation, or accidentally come across them during your journey. Situational awareness, having a response ready, and weighing your pros and cons are all ways you can quickly respond to triggering situations in which you may want to indulge in excess sugar.

TIP 1: Acknowledging Your Triggers

Without awareness, you can be caught off guard. By identifying and acknowledging what your triggers are early into your breakup with sugar, you can prepare yourself mentally and physically for when they come up in everyday life. Food for many of us means comfort, and by creating a new routine that brings the same comfort as a doughnut used to, for example, you don't have to go through the mental challenge of fighting off a trigger when it's in your environment.

TIP 2: Disassociation

Like I've previously said, food can be associated with comfort, memories, and peace in a time of chaos. Although this is an unhealthy way to cope, it could be the only way you knew how to. Instead, disassociating foods from "calming" feelings can allow you to establish new grounds. Over time, you'll form new memories and feelings that have nothing to do with food, but rather are about the people, places, and things you love! Not only can this allow you to leave sugar in the dust, but it can also bring new meaning to friendships, celebrations, and traditions. For example, your brain will now love the fact that you got to go on an evening walk with your partner, rather than driving to get ice cream.

TIP 3: Make a List of Pros and Cons

You've already made it this far, so why stop! When coming across triggers that could be a temptation, remind yourself of all the reasons you gave up sugar and how it has helped you live a better life. Creating a pros and cons list as to why you're giving up sugar can help put your mind back into a state where you are focusing on how you're improving your health and happiness and why you want to avoid triggers that may remind you how you used to eat or view sugar. For example, cutting back on sugar will help to improve your focus, which can make you feel more productive and organized. So next time you encounter a stressor and are leaning toward using sugar as a crutch, remember that doing so will take you further from your goals. When you see how much the pros of giving up sugar outweigh the cons (are there really any?), you'll find that the triggers will seem less powerful.

Sugar Withdrawal: What to Expect

Withdrawal symptoms from food addiction can be physical and psychological in nature. Research shows that humans who are addicted to refined foods report evidence of withdrawal when those foods are cut out. These withdrawal symptoms are often inevitable, and may include fatigue, irritability, sadness, lethargy, lack of interest in exercise, headaches, strong food cravings, and drowsiness. The good news is that withdrawal tends to be short-lived, and usually subsides within a week or two of changing your diet. But during your initial part of this journey of reducing your sugar intake, you may experience these physical and emotional symptoms that make it harder to resist high-sugar foods. At this point, it is vital to remind yourself that the strong desire to eat certain refined foods when abstaining from them is one of the main reasons you're hooked on sugar. It is a vicious cycle of bingeing, withdrawal, and craving that got you here in the first place, and now it's time to break that cycle.

As mentioned previously, irritability is a common withdrawal symptom within the first few weeks of sugar reduction. It's important to push past this irritability, and not give in to sugary snacks to make you temporarily feel better. Whenever withdrawal symptoms arise, recognizing them and knowing how to cope with the symptoms can make a big difference. Also, as you work through the steps in chapter 5, you'll find that slowly reducing your intake of sugars can lessen the withdrawal period and make symptoms less intense than if you were to quit cold turkey.

Coping with Withdrawal Symptoms

The withdrawal symptoms experienced when breaking sugar addiction can be intense for some people. How strongly you experience these symptoms will depend on how much sugar you've been consuming, and for how long. The key is not to be fooled by these symptoms and let them trick you into eating sugar to make you feel better (see p. 75 in chapter 3 about how addiction tricks our brains through the opponent-process cycle).

Think about this scenario: You are feeling lethargic. You think maybe your blood sugar is low and you grab a sugary granola bar to boost it back up. Guess what? You just got scammed by the sugar cycle. It is 99 percent likely that your blood sugar is just fine, and you are lethargic because it is part of the sugar withdrawal you are experiencing. Therefore, it's important to be aware of the symptoms of withdrawal so that you can properly attribute them to your situation when you're cutting back on added sugars.

The key to lessening withdrawal symptoms is to gradually reduce your intake of sugars. Research has shown that you are significantly more likely to succeed in reducing your sugar intake when you do so gradually. This can be beneficial to both lessening your symptoms and your overall health outcomes. Despite how difficult withdrawal symptoms make this process, there are things you can do to counter the strong urge to consume the foods you're trying to avoid.

TIP 1: Remember Your Long-Term Goal

Throughout this process, it is best to maintain focus on the long-term goal, instead of what's occurring at the moment. Withdrawal is difficult but will only be around for a short period of time (a few days or weeks, for most people, and studies show it usually peaks around days 2 to 5 after changing your diet). Oftentimes we must sacrifice immediate pleasure for rewards later. A technique commonly used when breaking addiction is to create a list that contains goals for implementing your plan. For example, one of your long-term goals for giving up sugar might be to lose weight to reduce your risk of diabetes and cardiovascular disease, so keep that goal (and how accomplished you'll feel when you reach it) in mind. Which would make you feel better: losing the weight you wanted, or having a pint of ice cream right now? The discomfort that comes from withdrawal is only temporary, and the key is not to lose sight of the long-term rewards that will come.

TIP 2: Rely on Your Support System

Another key to coping with withdrawal symptoms is to establish a strong support system. Discussing your journey with family and friends has been shown to be very important in the process of recovering from addiction. Support during withdrawal is particularly important to prevent relapses, and encouragement during this time is especially important when the urge comes to consume the foods you're trying to avoid. Overall, support from family and friends provides encouragement and can enhance your motivation to keep reaching your desired goals. However, sometimes it isn't always clear who is on your support "team." You might have the greatest friends and family in the world, but they might not be able to support you in the ways that you need. This often comes from their lack of taking your interest in cutting back on sugar seriously. They say "Just eat whatever you want, you look great!" and mean to be encouraging, but this type of language isn't going to support your goals. So be prepared to find support outside of your usual network if needed. This could be something more formal (like Overeaters Anonymous), or hiring a health coach or dietitian. Or it can be as simple as finding a friend of a friend who perhaps has also struggled with their diet in the past and would be willing to lend a sympathetic ear. Others who have gone through the process are often best able to support someone who is going through it because they can relate on a personal level and from their own experiences.

TIP 3: Practice Mindfulness

In addition to social support, practicing mindfulness can be helpful. For a long time, I was resistant to the idea that mindfulness could be beneficial, largely because I didn't understand what mindfulness actually is. It is essentially the art of stillness and focus, and comes in a variety of forms. You can practice mindfulness by sitting in a chair and just focusing on breathing, or petting your dog, or whatever singular task you want to devote your thoughts to. It can come in more formal avenues, through yoga or meditation techniques, which can be beneficial, especially for people who have a hard time being mindful without some guidance. Stretching and moving through yoga practices can stimulate blood flow, resulting in relieved tension and less muscle pain. Practicing mindfulness can enhance your ability to understand the emotional responses you may have during this period. Research shows that mindfulness meditations can be effective in lowering anxiety, physical pain, and depression—which are all common withdrawal symptoms.

The practice of being mindful can be very helpful when you're trying to distract yourself from sugar withdrawal symptoms, or when you're experiencing a craving. Focusing on something else can often be a way to allow you the time you need to distance yourself from the temporary negative thoughts linked to the addiction.

TIP 4: Plan Ahead

Although not everyone experiences withdrawal symptoms, it is beneficial to plan ahead in the event those moments do happen. Thinking of coping strategies for moments of withdrawal before they happen can prepare you to best deal with the situation. For example, instead of grabbing a packaged cookie for your snack when a craving arises, grab a handful of almonds or carrots or a piece of fruit (flip to pp. 171–178 for a list of some specific foods science tells us are great for combating sugar withdrawal). Planning for irritability could be as simple as purchasing a bath product for a relaxing soak in the tub.

Other examples are trying a new workout class or playing a game with your children. I can't stress enough the value of exercise and physical activity in the process of reducing your sugar intake. Not only does exercise release endorphins and other feel-good chemicals in your brain, but it also serves as a stress outlet and can help you relax. The goal is to have some ideas handy that will work for you if the moment strikes. If your withdrawal symptoms come hard and fast (a splitting headache, for example), you can treat the symptoms as you would if they arose in any other situation, such as with over-the-counter treatments (ibuprofen) for a headache. Lastly, don't forget about sleep. Going to bed early can be the best solution to coping with sugar withdrawal symptoms. When you're well rested, you will be better equipped the next day to manage your cravings.

TIP 5: Revise Your View of Reward

Most of us have been conditioned to associate highly processed foods that are high in sugar as a "reward." This situation is commonly referred to as the displaced reward-punishment syndrome. Behavior like this is reinforced at an early age with our parents stating, "If you eat your broccoli, you can have a piece of cake." From these early interactions, an idea is created that the healthy choice is a punishment and the unhealthy choice is a reward. This conditioned behavior can make its way into our daily lives, and we end up rewarding ourselves with foods that can be harmful to our bodies. By recognizing that, we can reverse this thinking and not succumb to sugar cravings.

Fortunately, there are some ways to overcome the displaced reward-punishment syndrome and move toward sustainable results. One way is to recognize that providing a reward of nutrient-poor food is backward thinking and not healthy for the body. Additionally, creating a list of your favorite healthy whole foods can help you rethink your rewards. This process involves changing your mindset and realizing that fueling your body with healthy foods is actually more rewarding than consuming those high-sugar options.

Curbing Cravings

As I discussed in chapter 3, cravings occur naturally in all human beings. Sometimes our body craves certain foods for biological reasons, such as having low blood sugar or being deficient in a specific micronutrient. Cravings can also be hedonic, meaning that foods are craved for the pleasure that is received from consuming them. Hedonic cravings explain why we crave things like chocolate and sweet foods so commonly—our brain remembers the pleasure those foods gave it.

Consuming excess sugary foods may alter the brain mechanisms that are responsible for processing rewards. Unfortunately, craving sugar is an inevitable component of kicking a sugar addiction. Conquering the symptoms of withdrawal and cravings can be rather difficult when dealing with sugar addiction. Although this is a normal part of the experience, there are some techniques you can implement that will help make this process more bearable. Let's talk about some now.

Use the Right Foods to Battle Your Cravings

When you have a craving, giving in to a sugary snack is not an option, but you may be able to help beat your craving by snacking on something else. Alternative food sources might satisfy your cravings and also benefit your health. Let's look at some of those options.

Eat High-Protein Foods

High-protein foods are an excellent way to reduce and satisfy sugar cravings when they arise. Foods that are high in protein typically contain very little sugar content. Since high-protein foods like seafood, chicken, nuts, whole fruits, vegetables, and eggs contain such a high amount of protein, they are more satiating.

Satiety occurs when the body feels full and satisfied; consuming high-protein foods will allow the body to feel full for a longer period of time. The idea behind consuming high-protein foods in place of sugary foods is that it eliminates the urge to overindulge. Since chicken, beef, fish, and eggs keep your body feeling satisfied, you're not eating these foods for hedonic pleasure.

High-protein food sources supply the body with many nutrients, including protein, niacin, thiamin, riboflavin, vitamin B-6, vitamin E, iron, zinc, and magnesium. It's important to recognize that when eating protein-rich sources, we consider the protein "package." The idea behind the protein package is that whenever we consume protein, we are often also getting fat, fiber, sodium, and even more. This protein package is likely to make a difference to our health.

For example, 1 cup of cooked lentils not only provides the body with 18 g of protein, but also 15 g of fiber. Lentils also contain no saturated fat or sodium. Consuming protein-rich foods keeps us fuller longer, and they are also packed with nutrients that can benefit our health.

Chicken. A medium piece of grilled chicken breast provides the body with 17.8 g of protein, along with various other essential vitamins and minerals. For example, grilled chicken breast contains 16.8 mg of magnesium, 211 mg of potassium, 18 µg of selenium, and 4.2 µg of folate. Chicken is known as a complete protein, which means it provides the body with all nine essential amino acids.

Seafood. One medium salmon fillet that is baked can provide the body with 58.6 g of protein. It also provides the body with 20.4 g of calcium, 1,050 mg of potassium, 10.7 µg of vitamin B-12, and 90.8 µg of vitamin A. Salmon is also a great source of omega-3 fatty acids. The amount of omega-3 fatty acids that each fish provides depends on the foods they are fed, but on average, salmon can provide the body with brain-nourishing omega-3 fatty acids (1.24 g of DHA and 0.58 g of EPA).

Eggs. Two scrambled eggs provide the body with 12.5 g of protein. Eggs are another complete protein that provide the body with various micronutrients. Two eggs contain 56 mg of calcium, 35 µg of folate, 2 µg of vitamin D, 0.433 mg of riboflavin, and 1.28 mg of zinc. Eggs are packed with vitamins and minerals and promote the feeling of fullness due to their high protein content.

Nuts. Although considered incomplete proteins—they do not provide the body with all nine amino acids—nuts still contain most of the essential ones. About 1 cup of unshelled pistachios contains 26.1 g of protein. One cup also contains 12.8 g of fiber, 1,250 mg of potassium, 5 mg of iron, 582 mg of phosphorus, 2.91 mg of zinc, 1.7 mg of niacin, and 3.71 mg of vitamin C. There are a variety of nuts to choose from that leave the body feeling full and nourished, such as peanuts, cashews, Brazil nuts, macadamia nuts, walnuts, and pecans.

Vegetables. There are plenty of vegetables that provide the body with protein and promote fullness. For example, 1 cup of raw green peas can provide the body with 7.86 g of protein. Peas also contain 2.13 mg of iron, 354 mg of potassium, 36.2 mg of calcium, 2.61 µg of vitamin C, and 3.03 mg of niacin. Broccoli is another option—1 cup of chopped broccoli has 2.6 g of protein and also provides over 100 percent of your daily need for vitamins C and K.

What about fruits? I'll talk about the benefits that fruits can have in the next section, but when it comes to protein, fruits tend to be lower in it than vegetables, nuts, and legumes.

Naturally Sweet Fruits

A sugar craving can be satisfied by foods other than carbohydrates and added sugars. Fruits are a natural source of sugar that can alleviate a sugar craving. Fruits vary in how sweet they are, but each contains additional benefits that make them the advantageous choice over added sugars.

Fruits are rich sources of fiber, antioxidants, vitamins, and minerals, all of which are important in fighting your sugar cravings. Fiber helps keep you feeling full, decreasing the amount and how often one eats. In addition, fiber helps maintain healthy bowel movements, reducing any digestion problems. Antioxidants help neutralize free radicals. Free radicals can damage cells in the body, leading to conditions such as cancer. Antioxidants prevent free radicals from doing so, decreasing one's risk for developing such conditions. Polyphenols are another compound found in fruit that contribute to its benefits. Polyphenols protect cells against ultraviolet radiation and pathogens. Research suggests a diet rich in plant polyphenols can help prevent the development of a plethora of diseases, such as cancer, osteoporosis, cardiovascular disease, diabetes, and neurodegenerative diseases.

Vitamins and minerals each have various properties that help the body maintain optimal health. Vitamin C, a common vitamin found in fruits, helps boost the body's immune system and build collagen, which is essential for strong connective tissue in the body. Potassium works in opposition to sodium, helping to lower blood pressure, reducing one's risk for hypertension, stroke, and cardiovascular disease. The B vitamins, including niacin, thiamin, and riboflavin, all aid in energy production. Maintaining B vitamins is essential to ensuring normal energy reactions and energy levels.

The twelve sweetest fruits (in order of sweetness) are grapes, cherries, mangos, bananas, apples, pears, kiwi, pineapple, plums, peaches, oranges, and apricots. Keep these on hand, and think about ways to incorporate them into your diet to help you manage your sugar cravings.

#1 Grapes.

One cup has 21 percent daily value (DV) of copper, 18 percent DV of vitamin K, and 8 percent DV of riboflavin. It also contains 1.4 g of fiber, which accounts for about 6 percent of the recommended fiber intake. Helps maintain healthy blood pressure and reduces cholesterol.

#2 Cherries.

One cup has 3.15 g of dietary fiber, aiding in keeping you full and satiated, plus 18 percent DV of vitamin C, 10 percent DV of potassium, and 5 percent DV of copper. Rich source of antioxidants. Can improve sleep quality by increasing melatonin.

#3 Mangos.

Contains 67 percent DV of vitamin C, 20 percent DV of copper, and 18 percent DV of folate. Mango also has lutein and zeaxanthin, two antioxidants that have been shown to protect the eyes against damage from blue light.

#4 Bananas.

One banana contains 12 percent DV of vitamin C, 11 percent DV of copper, 10 percent DV of potassium, and 3 g of fiber, 12 percent of the recommended intake. Can help enhance digestion and improve gastrointestinal health.

#5 Apples.

One medium apple has 25 percent DV of fiber, 10 percent DV of vitamin C, and 5 percent DV of potassium. Polyphenols in apples can help reduce cardiovascular disease risk. Polyphenols also have anticancer and antiviral properties and protect against Alzheimer's disease.

#6 Pears.

A medium pear has 16 percent DV of copper, 12 percent DV of vitamin C, and 5 percent DV of vitamin K. Rich source of antioxidants and contains anthocyanins, which can possibly lower risk for type 2 diabetes.

#7 Kiwi.

One kiwi has 62 percent DV of vitamin C, 23 percent DV of vitamin K, and 5 percent DV of potassium, as well as 2.1 g of fiber, 8 percent of the recommended intake. Has the antioxidants lutein and zeaxanthin, which protect eyes from blue light. Helps promote regular bowel movements.

#8 Pineapple.

One cup of pineapple has 131 percent DV of vitamin C, 76 percent DV of manganese, and 9 percent DV of vitamin B6. Contains bromelain, which helps with relieving osteoarthritis and diarrhea and increases the absorption of antibiotics. Bromelain has also been found to have anticancerous properties as it promotes cell death.

#9 Plums.

One plum contains 10 percent DV of vitamin C, 5 percent DV of vitamin A, and 3 percent DV of potassium. It has antioxidant, anti-inflammatory, and antiallergic properties that are associated with improved bone health, cognitive function, and reduced cardiovascular risk factors.

#10 Peaches.

One peach has 17 percent DV of vitamin C, 10 percent DV of vitamin A, and 8 percent DV of potassium. Peaches improve water retention and skin moisture.

#11 Oranges.

One orange has 95 percent DV of vitamin C, 10 percent DV of fiber, and 9 percent DV of folate. Contains the compounds hesperidin and naringenin. Hesperidin has been found to reduce systolic blood pressure and pulse in individuals with hypertension. Naringenin has been found to improve cells that line the inside of blood vessels.

#12 Apricots.

Two apricots have 8 percent DV of vitamin C, 4 percent DV of vitamin E, and potassium. Vitamin C and vitamin E both promote eye health.

Stock Your Kitchen with Craving Crushers

Focusing on high-protein foods and sweeter fruits, like the ones I recommend above, can be a great asset to helping cope with your sugar cravings. But I have more secret hacks for you to battle those cravings! There are some specific foods that have been shown to help reduce sugar cravings. You're going to want to stock up on these and keep them handy. The good news is that none of these are fancy. They're all readily available at a supermarket.

Craving Crusher #1: Berries

Yes, berries are a fruit, but they get their own category because they crush your cravings not due to their sweetness, but to other benefits they provide. Berries contain a ton of fiber and are considered low GI. This in turn creates a low-level insulin spike compared to other fruits that contain high sugar content. Including berries in your meals and dishes can help curb a natural sweet tooth. Berries also have a high water content when compared to other fruits and can aid in hydration. Finally, berries contain polyphenols. Polyphenols have been linked to decreasing inflammation in the gut lining, which can be harmed through sugar addiction and keep people addicted. By decreasing this inflammation, you can overcome a sugar craving and, further down the line, a sugar addiction. Including berries in things like homemade sauces, unsweetened iced tea, or as a fun yogurt bowl topping can help you stay hydrated and kick your cravings. Also, check out the recipes for Blueberry Oatmeal Muffins (p. 260), Frozen Yogurt Bark with Nuts and Berries (p. 257), and Strawberry Shortcake Parfait (p. 255), which include berries.

Craving Crusher #2: Avocados

Avocados, like berries, get their own category as a standout fruit because they have proven that the combination of fat and fiber can also be a hunger-crusher. In a clinical trial, avocados were substituted for carbohydrate-dense, low-fat breakfast ingredients. The trial found that the satiety hormones in the brain were more prevalent after consuming the avocado versus the high-carb meal. This can prevent sugar cravings by reducing the overall feelings of hunger. We don't crave something sweet when we are fully nourished by monounsaturated fats and fiber—found in avocado! Not an avocado fan? Try blending them into a pesto, smoothie, or dressing to get a creamy texture and all of the benefits. Avocados are in a few of the recipes I've developed for you—check out the Coconut Avocado Lime Soup (p. 228), Chickpea-Avocado Sandwich (p. 235), and Stuffed Avocados (p. 237).

Craving Crusher #3: Pistachios

For decades, it has been known that nut consumption can help improve our health, including lowering cardiometabolic markers and BMI. Pistachios can therefore displace the need for sweets and promote an overall healthy dietary pattern. They're packed with protein, which is an important factor when addressing sugar addiction. Protein is made up of amino acids, which can build the pathways in our brain that stop sugar addiction. When the neurotransmitter levels and hormones in the brain are functioning properly, they will be deterred from wanting unhealthy food options, like soda and candy. A recent study showed that regular pistachio consumption was associated with weight loss and other cardiometabolic health benefits, including lower blood pressure, and best of all, it was also shown to reduce intake of sweets! So, grab a handful of pistachios next time you feel a sugar craving coming on, or build your own sugar-free trail mix using pistachios and other on-the-go foods such as cacao nibs. They are also a recommended nut in my Frozen Yogurt Bark in the recipe section (p. 257)!

Craving Crusher #4: Chia Seeds

Chia seeds are full of essential fatty acids that fuel our body and its pathways. They are also a complete plant protein, containing all nine essential amino acids. This is important because it means these seeds are of high biological value (HBV). HBV proteins are easier for our bodies to absorb and utilize, and therefore control sugar cravings. Finally, chia seeds have a lipid profile that has been proven to prevent blood glucose spikes and improve blood lipid profiles. This can also benefit those with a sugar addiction because of the long-lasting effects chia seeds have on the entire body, not just one area or system. Chia seeds are a great way to sneak up on a craving. Sprinkling them on top of toasted bread with a little cream cheese, in oatmeal, or all alone in chia pudding can taste great and stop cravings in their tracks. Chia seeds are an ingredient in the Sugarless Granola at the end of the book (p. 218).

Craving Crusher #5: Chickpeas

Legumes in general are a staple in the diets of some of the healthiest populations worldwide, including the Mediterranean. Legumes are filled with fiber and plant-based protein. The overall nutritional components of chickpeas make them a great choice for overcoming sugar addiction. They have little flavor and are very versatile, while still packing a total of 18 to 22 g of fiber per 100 g of chickpeas! Fiber is split into insoluble and soluble categories. Chickpeas contain both kinds of fiber, making them beneficial to the overall gut microbiome diversification. Having a diverse gut microbiome can improve cravings along the gut-brain connection and signal hunger and fullness to the brain at a more efficient rate. If you're looking for some delicious chickpea recipes to get you started, check out the Chickpea-Avocado Sandwich (p. 235), Olive Hummus (p. 266), and Old Bay® Roasted Chickpeas (p. 246). Don't be afraid to get creative by swapping other ingredients out for chickpeas, like pizza dough ingredients and sauce!

Craving Crusher #6: Oats

Oats are a whole-grain powerhouse. They contain fast-digesting and slow-digesting carbohydrates that provide your body with a boost of energy and prevent fatigue. Fatigue is one of the leading causes of sugar cravings. When we are tired, our body craves fast-digesting energy (like sugar). Oats, however, can benefit our bodies much more than sugar can. Oats contain a soluble dietary fiber called beta-glucan. Beta-glucan has been shown to reduce postprandial (after feeding) glucose values as well as cholesterol. This can help our bodies break away from sugar addiction and maintain a healthy biochemical state. Oats can be added to many different meals to replace white flour! Thicken up a sauce or stew using oat flour, by blending oats in your blender or food processor until fine. Try making Sugarless Granola (p. 218), Oatmeal Breakfast Cookies (p. 223), and Blueberry Oatmeal Muffins (p. 260), which all use oats.

Craving Crusher #7: Olives

Polyunsaturated fatty acids (PUFA) found in olives when combined with carbohydrate intake have been shown to regulate our glucose-insulin homeostasis. But how is this important when trying to break a sugar addiction? Our bodies utilize glucose as our main energy source. While glucose is a good thing to have around, glucose that lingers in our bloodstream is problematic. Insulin comes in to help by signaling to the body that it's time to absorb the glucose from our blood into our cells. Homeostasis between these mechanisms is crucial when evaluating insulin resistance, which is a common condition among those who consume too much sugar in their diets. PUFAs are also beneficial for heart health and overall longevity! Think tapenades, cheese boards, and salad additive to spice up your meals using olives. They're a great snack, or check out the Flaxseed Crackers and Olive Hummus recipe (p. 266), which uses olives.

Craving Crusher #8: Sweet Potatoes

Sweet potatoes have almost the same macronutrients as regular white potatoes, but they stand out because of their micronutrient content. Sweet potatoes contain an inactive form of vitamin A known as carotenoids. Carotenoids have the power to improve our cognitive function over time. They can also prevent diseases of lifestyle, including eye issues and cancer, but the real sugar rewiring power they hold comes from our brains. Our brains utilize neuro-stimulation and hormones to affect our mood and daily function. Sugar stimulates dopamine, or the happy neurochemical. Vitamin A can help combat this by reducing sugar cravings and regulating the release of dopamine. Sweet potatoes are an easy side dish when baked, or a vehicle for protein. Keeping roasted sweet potatoes prepared for a week's worth of meals can save you time and sugar cravings.

Craving Crusher #9: Greek Yogurt

Unsweetened Greek yogurt is packed with protein and a great replacement for normally high-fat condiments and ingredients like sour cream. The protein in Greek yogurt is a complete protein and is known for keeping us satiated for long periods of time and therefore prevents sugar binges at night. One meta-analysis looked at the effects of protein on appetite and found that meals containing complete proteins increase fullness ratings more than lower-protein meals. This, in turn, influences BMI and metabolic syndrome. Incorporating more Greek yogurt into your cooking can allow for less sugar in the long run. A go-to snack can be fresh veggie dip using Greek yogurt and seasonings. Check out the Eggy Roasted Red Pepper Wraps (p. 221) and the Sugarless Ranch Dip (p. 253), which use Greek yogurt.

Craving Crusher #10: Spirulina

Spirulina is a nutritional powerhouse alga that is dried into a bright green powder for consumption. It contains multiple vitamins and minerals, and there is also evidence to support its role in reducing appetite and blood lipid levels. Spirulina was used in a placebo-controlled study to see its effect on appetite and lipid profiling. The findings showed significant reduced appetite when the participants consumed 1 g per day of spirulina in their diets. By reducing over-all appetite, your body no longer craves the high blood glucose spike that is satisfied by sugary foods and the uncontrollable eating aspects sugar gives to food, and therefore you won't feel the need to consume sugar! You can add some spirulina to your smoothie for a boost of nutrition and a little help with lessening those sugar cravings. You can also disguise spirulina in spreads such as mashed avocado, and condiments such as mayo and ketchup!

▶●◀

Making the decision to give up added sugar and replace it with craving-crushing foods can be a simple thought, but in the end there are many triggers and other outstanding factors that affect the way our brain works—even without the sugar! Choosing foods to curb cravings and knowing the signs of sugar withdrawal can help immensely. But there are inevitable situations that arise that can derail our sugar-skipping efforts. The next chapter will help you dive deep into the three S's: stressors, setbacks, and social pressures.

CHAPTER 6

HOW TO MANAGE THE THREE *S*'S: STRESSORS, SETBACKS, AND SOCIAL PRESSURES

Now that you know the steps you need to take on your sugar-less journey, you are well on your way to succeeding at changing your life for the better. But it won't always be easy. Knowing what to do, and actually doing it, takes a lot of work and effort, but remember this: the secret to success is in not allowing day-to-day living to move you away from your health goals. Certain challenges that we all encounter can threaten to do this if you aren't ready for them. In this chapter, I'll review some ways in which you can combat the three biggest challenges that people typically face when trying to reduce their sugar: stress, setbacks, and social pressures. I've touched on each of these topics throughout the book, but here I want to offer some specific tips and guidance to help you in the likely event that you encounter these issues.

Managing Stress

We all have stress. We're supposed to. We need stress to help us survive in the world, and without it we wouldn't live very long. Our brains were built to take on stressors in our environment and "fight" them or take "flight" and get out of the way. This "fight-or-flight" response is an evolutionary adaptive feature that we've all inherited. Back when we were hunters and gatherers, we may have encountered life-threatening stressors regularly—such as coming face to face with a bear. This stressor (the bear) provokes a series of events in our brains and bodies to give us the energy and willpower to fight, or to flee.

Like our caveman ancestors, we encounter stressors all the time and react in ways that allow us to deal with the situation and essentially survive it. The problem nowadays is that for most of us, our daily stressors aren't life-threatening, but our brains are still acting like they are. Under chronic stress from work, family life, social pressures, financials concerns, etc., we are stressed out, and most of the time we don't deal with it appropriately. As discussed in chapter 4, stress can have an impact on our food choices, and in many cases, we use it as a way to "self-medicate" when minor (or major) stressors occur in life. Why do we do this? Because it works. If you're feeling overwhelmed by your to-do list, the dopamine rush from a sugary snack will improve how you feel in the moment, and make that endless to-do list feel a bit more manageable. Evidence shows that when people are stressed, they consume high fat and sugary foods more frequently. A cycle emerges in which stress stimulates the hormone cortisol, and cortisol stimulates appetite. In times of stress, these highly palatable comfort foods provide us with a sense of pleasure or distract us from the stress.

The way to make sure that you're not letting stress dictate your diet is to ensure you are properly evaluating your stressors. In most cases, we're "stressing" about things that really are no threat to us. It is all about our *appraisal* of the stressors. Let me explain more.

When we encounter a stressor of any kind, we have a *primary* appraisal of it. This is a very quick mental reaction in which we decide if this stressor is really an immediate threat to us. So, for example, if you get an email on the weekend from your boss with the subject line "URGENT," you might make the primary appraisal that this is a potential stressor.

However, we need more information than that to make a realistic appraisal of whether our stressors are significant. That's where the *secondary appraisal* comes in. This is the part where we think for a second about the context and our past experiences. If you're in charge of a huge project at work that was due on Friday, and you never get emails from your boss, let alone ones titled "URGENT,"

SHOULD I GET MY CORTISOL LEVELS CHECKED?

Since we know that cortisol is linked to stress and appetite, you might be wondering if you should get yours measured to see if it's out of whack. You can purchase tests online, and while cortisol tests are offered in labs, doctors typically only prescribe them to rule out certain diseases or conditions. Should you do it? My take on it is no. Cortisol levels are dynamic and change throughout the day. This is why if you want to tell whether you're "stressed," you can't simply go get your cortisol levels checked. They will fluctuate throughout the day. You're better off taking steps to reduce stress in your life and learning how to manage it better—then your cortisol levels will eventually be where they should be.

you may correctly assume something is up and you might correctly start to feel stressed. But if instead your boss is throwing a surprise birthday party that evening for your coworker, you might assume that the email is related to the party, and you wouldn't see it as a huge threat. Or, if your boss has the habit of sending out funny memes over email and does this often on the weekends, you might assume this is another joke she's passing along.

When you encounter a stressor, it is vital to pause and reflect before you react and allow the stress to mount. Many times, we stress about stuff that, when put into context, isn't really stressful—but we are letting it be!

Tips for Managing Stress without Turning to Sugar

TIP 1: Increase Your Physical Activity

Exercising may be a helpful way to prevent eating a lot of sugar when you're feeling the sudden urge to indulge in response to a stressor. One study found that people who were highly active chose healthier foods when coping with stress. Not to say they didn't also reach for energy-dense foods as well (they still indulged in sweets from time to time), but their overall diet consisted of more fruits and veggies compared to those who were less active. Even if adopting physical activity into your routine doesn't impact your veggie choices, it can be a way to handle outside stressors instead of reaching for sugar. Although working out when feeling stressed might be lowest on your list of things you want to do, it has been shown to elevate one's mood and may lessen the way you perceive stress, while improving quality of life. Since mood and dietary behaviors are so closely related, doing a quick ten-minute routine is more helpful than it sounds. Furthermore, people who exercise regularly have less cortisol secreted after a psychological stressor compared to those who exercise less. If you're someone who eats out of boredom at the end of the day, and not because of stress, physical activity is an excellent distraction. If you find you're more bored at night, maybe try a nighttime exercise routine. If doing a high-intensity workout at night isn't for you, maybe just going for a walk is enough of a distraction to prevent a sugar lapse.

TIP 2: Promote Positive Relationships

Communication is key in dealing with any stressors, especially when you used to turn to eating sugar. When reviewing our ways of communication with ourselves and our loved ones, it's important to first recognize why you've turned to food instead of a friend to begin with! Things like calling a friend to just chat, or communicating with your partner, not only help decompress feelings of stress and reduce cortisol levels, but can also distract us from trying to eat sugary comfort foods. It has been shown in teens with poor friendships that their body dissatisfaction and eating behaviors were also altered, making their stress levels a lot higher (and continuing the cycle). By creating meaningful relationships based in positivity and support, you will be successful in your no-sugar journey.

TIP 3: Learn Other Behaviors to Cope

Eating sugar as a habit doesn't align with your current health goals, so finding alternatives to cope with stress outside of eating can be extremely beneficial to your mental well-being. There have been many studies done on food patterns and healthy eating in relation to mindfulness activities. What is a mindfulness activity, you may ask? These practices can include anything from breathwork, stretching, meditation, or journaling, to things like doing a jigsaw or word puzzle, sewing, making crafts, or cleaning. It's more about keeping your mind occupied and your hands busy than it is about what activity you do. Scientists have found that meditation and mindfulness training have helped many in preventing binges on unhealthy foods, and overall support a healthy lifestyle free of emotional eating. When these practices become part of your daily routine, they turn into a more satisfying habit for our brains to focus on than stress-eating sugar! Just like sugar can give us a dopamine rush, so can yoga.

TIP 4: Get a Quality Night's Sleep

Sleep is tied to so many aspects of our health, including our stress levels. Getting the proper amount of quality sleep every night (meaning deep sleep) allows our bodies to feel energized and ready to take on another day without sugar. Sugar, as we've talked about before, is a source of quick energy and is often craved when we don't get enough sleep at night. By losing sleep, you could also be at risk for other lifestyle diseases . . . and pairing this with poor eating behaviors triggered by poor sleep means chaos! And you don't want something like sleep to knock you off your no-sugar track. There are many tools you can use to ensure you get enough sleep every night. Avoiding eating two to three hours before bedtime, discontinuing the use of electronics before bedtime, and wearing blue light protective glasses when looking at screens for long periods of time throughout the day can all help improve your sleep and therefore reduce stress and help you avoid sugar. Sugar is disruptive to your sleep, so making the change to a sugarless diet will have the added advantage of helping you to rest better at night and feel bright-eyed in the morning.

Managing Setbacks

If you recall, I said back in chapter 4 that "life is not linear." There are bound to be points in time where we have setbacks, whether that's in our career, our relationships, or even in our health.

As much as you think you have complete control of what you eat in any given day, when you take a closer look, you start to realize that sometimes the decision is already made for you. And if *you* aren't making the decision about what you eat, then who the heck is? The food environment!

It's no wonder that the food environment has been blamed for the obesity epidemic. Thanks to our current food environment, which is inundated with ultra-processed foods that are high in calories and sugar, dietary lapses and setbacks are very common among people who are trying to avoid sugar. Initially, you might think that your food environment only includes what you physically have available to you—whether it's a convenience store where you can grab a snack, a restaurant close to your job that you order from for lunch, or a small grocery store versus a large chain where you do most of your grocery shopping. However, the physical environment is only one

MAKING SENSE OF SETBACKS

I prefer the term *setback*, but this generally refers to what others may call *lapses* and *relapses*. It's important to note the difference between these terms. A lapse is considered a temporary slip, whereas a relapse is a deterioration after a period of improvement and a return to the former state. In other words, a lapse would be like having a doughnut for breakfast but moving past it and getting right back on track, whereas a relapse would be allowing that one doughnut to translate into throwing in the towel and just going back to your old ways of eating. People lapse and relapse for a variety of different reasons. Negative emotions and stress are common triggers, as is being in "high-risk" situations that threaten your sense of control. High-risk situations can be anything from walking past your favorite bakery to bringing a tub of ice cream into your house. While there's no way to completely avoid external triggers, learning how to identify them and self-regulate your response is vital in preventing a lapse from snowballing into a relapse.

part of our food environment. Affordability, convenience, desirability, and availability all make up our food environment. Our sociocultural surroundings, opportunities, nutrient quality, national policy, and economics impact these aspects as well. Since the components of one's food environment are so closely intertwined, if we reach for something high in sugar, it's apparent that it's not only because of a lapse in our own willpower.

TIP 1: Keep Track of What You Eat and How You Feel

When you hear the term *emotional eating*, it's important to keep in mind that it's not always in response to negative emotions. Indeed, people also turn to food when they are happy. Taking note of when you find yourself emotionally eating is the first step in working to prevent a future sugar lapse and home in on potential triggers for you. Although it can be time-consuming and feel like an annoying chore, writing down what you eat and the current mood you find yourself in has been shown to be helpful. Findings from dieting literature suggest that self-monitoring is vital to prevent a diet relapse. People who lost weight and maintained it were more likely to keep track of what they ate during the day as well as recognizing specific times when a lapse is more common. Tackle negative emotions and emotional eating head on by actively working to recognize them. Although this is easier said than done, it's an important first step. If you find that you turn to food as soon as you get upset, it's important to work to break that cycle. Try to swap out food for an activity, or call a close friend or family member. If you're not one who likes to share how they are feeling with others, try writing or journaling so you get it off your chest.

TIP 2: Don't Bring It in the House

Not having sugary favorites available in your fridge removes the temptation, because chances are you're not going to run out and get it the second the craving hits. This may be difficult for people who are impulse grocery shoppers, so if that's you, making an itemized list for the upcoming week instead of winging it is essential. However, if you didn't find time to make a list before running to the store, try to stay around the perimeter of the supermarket. Most of the sugar that lurks in our processed food is located on the aisles in the middle of the store, e.g., cereals, prepackaged cakes and crackers, and condiments. Although it's not always the case, the perimeter of most grocery stores is where you'll find the produce and protein-rich foods and less of the sugary beverages and chips.

But what do you do if you can't keep it out of the house, like if you have a roommate who says they are keeping their cookies on the premises, no matter what? In this case, I'd suggest creating some rules regarding the cabinet and refrigerator space. Perhaps your roommate could have their own shelf (preferably up high, or out of your immediate eyesight) that is just for *their* food, and off-limits to you (and vice versa). That way, you have some barrier to giving in and grabbing their stash when you have a craving.

Tip 3: Enlist a Support System (at Home and at Work)

People who actively make healthier behavior changes often find it helpful to enlist the support of close family and friends. In fact, social environment has been shown to be more influential on healthy eating than physical food environment. Whether this is because you have someone to help with food planning and prep, or someone whom you can turn to for encouragement, having the support of other people can help keep you on track. Another effective way to prevent setbacks is to avoid sugar with someone instead of on your own, such as your partner or a friend. Diet-specific social support has been shown to be more helpful in making healthful changes than going without specific support. This can help make mundane tasks more fun. Going food shopping, cooking a meal, or doing a new exercise class together makes healthful changes less daunting.

TIP 4: Plan Your Meals (All of Them)

Many of us are busier than we've ever been, and it feels like time is always running out. Studies have found that when working outside the home (which many do), food prep ultimately decreases, and the demand for convenience foods and takeout increases. This has become detrimental to our health because those of us who eat more than five meals at home per week are less likely to be overweight or obese and have a lower percentage of body fat compared to those who eat fewer than three meals per week at home. Unfortunately, it has been estimated that in some places people eat 30 to 40 percent of their calories from convenience foods and foods outside the home.

That's where planning in advance comes in. Although it's easier to grab a quick bite when you're on the go, chances are whatever you would have prepped at home is healthier than what's available to you while out. Bringing your own food to work or certain social settings can be helpful in situations where you're inundated with high-sugar foods. For example, if the break room at work always has snacks out in the open, make sure you bring your own from home so you're not tempted to grab a candy bar. Meal prepping can also be a game changer. If you know you're going to be getting home late several nights in the upcoming week, having something ready in advance takes all the guessing and scrambling out of mealtime when you're short on time. If you're prepping something that freezes well, make a couple of extra portions for a later date (and if you want some great freezer recipes to get you started, check out Blueberry Oatmeal Muffins (p. 260), Coconut Avocado Lime Soup (p. 228), or Eggy Roasted Red Pepper Wraps (p. 221). In general, saucy foods (like chili) and soups are great candidates because when reheated, they won't dry out. Homemade burgers (veggie or meat), baked falafel, and certain Crock-Pot® meals are other low-sugar meal ideas that defrost nicely as well. If you're not really into cooking, having bags of frozen vegetables on hand is an easy way to fill your plate with greens and not have to think about washing, dicing, and cooking anything beforehand. If you're not one for reheated food, have some easy meal ideas ready to go for those hectic nights. Frittatas, bagged salad mixes (not the ones with sugary dried fruits and dressings) with a can of tuna or salmon for protein, or steamed Chinese takeout are all fast, low-sugar ideas.

TIP 5: Accept Setbacks and Move On

Despite all the planning and best intentions, 99.9 percent of people experience some type of dietary setback, so chances are you will, too. However, don't view this as a failure. Remember that setbacks are just temporary. You may have not felt like you had a choice when they occur, but you do have a choice on whether you'll let a setback be what it is—a temporary thing—or allow it to derail you entirely.

From the start of your sugar-free journey, it is extremely important to set realistic expectations. Maintaining a diet low in sugar is going to be a challenge and you likely will lapse here and there. However, it's how you handle and move past the lapse that matters. If you chose to avoid sugar for weight-loss purposes, keep in mind that there is often a disconnect between expectations for weight-loss success and reality. The first thing to do is make sure not to beat yourself up over it and view the slipup as a failure. Instead, consider it a learning experience so you can better cope next time you find yourself in a similar situation. However, if you start feeling negatively about what happened, it can be a good idea to write it down or talk to someone about it. You don't want to internalize it and make the little blip bigger than it is. Sometimes, talking it through with someone can help you see that it isn't as big a deal as you're making it, and you can rally and move past it.

It's also important to try to pinpoint what triggered you to have a temporary lapse. Was it the people you were with, or were you alone? Was it your mood? Was it because you brought the food you shouldn't eat into the house and found it too hard to resist? Once you determine the trigger, you can plan better next time. If you feel like a lapse is going to turn into a relapse, start keeping track of what you're eating in greater detail and jot down your mood as well. Self-monitoring is one method that's been shown to be an effective strategy to stay on track and allows you to reflect on past lapses and plan for the next high-risk situation that could potentially trigger a sugar slip.

Surviving Social Pressures

Social pressures can come in many different forms. First, let's talk about the more recent type of social pressure that we've been grappling with: the internet.

As noted earlier, we really don't have complete control of the foods we put in our mouths. Besides our food environment, both social and mainstream media influence our choices as well. It's hard to remember a time when most people weren't glued to their phones at all hours of the day. Whether you're aimlessly scrolling on social media or reading news articles, you'll likely view countless pictures and articles centered on different foods and dietary topics. Healthy

foods, fast foods, gluten-free foods, "diet" foods, high-protein foods—
you name it, there's a post about it. In fact, after selfies, food photos
are the second most popular topic on Instagram. In addition, popular social media personalities, or "influencers," sometimes team up
with food advertisers to promote food products. Since social media is
so prominent in our lives, researchers have begun to study the relationship between social media and our own food choices. Recent
studies found that both Facebook and Instagram have been shown
to influence unhealthy food choices as well as overeating and body
dissatisfaction. Collectively, food photography, endless advertisements, and seeing your favorite influencer or others within your
social network promote (or eat) certain foods can lead to increased
intention to purchase and eat those same foods.

Although "influencers" in some cases can improve the positive attitude and purchasing intention of healthy foods, the majority of food posts highlight unhealthy foods. One recent study found
that advertisements on social media for unhealthy foods elicit a
more positive response from viewers compared to healthy foods.
The authors also found that participants were more likely to recall
unhealthy food brands they were exposed to in advertising as well
as want to "share" an unhealthy food post. Besides influencers,
celebrity accounts are also at fault for promoting junk foods, and
not only due to sponsorships. In fact, most posts aren't sponsored,
further reinforcing unhealthy dietary behaviors as a cultural norm.
Although much of the social media data comes out of the adolescent

literature, we have to wonder if it has a similar effect on adults. Unfortunately, many social media platforms have no restrictions on advertisements for junk foods, which is extremely problematic since social media is one of the preferred places to market. In addition, unhealthy food advertising in mainstream media is a continued public health problem. On any given day we are bombarded with advertisements promoting sugar-laden foods and drinks from multiple media outlets.

Food Porn

We also need to be aware of another form of social pressure that isn't always so obvious: food porn. You know what I mean—those innocent-seeming videos and images of gooey brownies fresh out of the oven that you can practically smell through your phone, or the slow addition of decadent toppings to a mountain of ice cream that makes you want to run out and buy all those ingredients. It isn't a coincidence that there are tons and tons of these videos online—people watch them, and just like watching sexual porn can arouse some people, watching food porn can arouse hunger. The science confirms this: in a recent study, people who showed greater brain activation in response to food images than erotic porn images were more likely to overeat. So it's a good idea to comb through your social media accounts and unfollow food-focused accounts that are known to post videos and photos of desserts and other treats that you're trying to avoid.

The Movie Made Me Eat It

Commercials zooming in on the crunchy ridges of the newest chip or the individual bubbles in a glass of soda make these same foods you try to avoid seem irresistible. And while television commercials are a popular avenue to advertise, foods aren't always promoted in such an obvious way, and can be hidden in plain view. Ultra-processed foods and drinks are often embedded in the story line of a television show or movie. In fact, over the last twenty-four years, diets in movies averaged a 16.5 percent higher sugar content per 2,000 calories than the average US citizen actually consumes. And although only around 12 percent of foods depicted in movies were branded, snacks like Lay's® chips and Hostess® pastries were clearly advertised. (Beverages like Coca-Cola® and Pepsi® are the most popular brands shown in movies.) Lastly, with the major shift from print to online news giving people constant access to the latest information, this is just another avenue for companies to promote their newest products, ultimately influencing behaviors. Taken together, it's easy to see that it's a lot more than just our physical location that makes up our food environment, and why almost everyone encounters some sort of dietary setback when trying to cut out sugar.

Sugar Pushers

In addition to the web-based social pressure many of us are exposed to when it comes to food, we also must cope with social pressures in real-life situations. Oftentimes the people in our life make it hard for us to stay on track. If your friends, family, and coworkers typically gravitate to sugary foods and ordering out, it's easy to save your prepped lunch for the next day and order in with the group. Even if it's not the intention of your friends and family to be a negative influence on your dietary goals, they exert influence over your attitudes and behavior. While this isn't the case for everyone you associate with, there is evidence to suggest that best friends and same-sex friends can potentially influence your weight. If your friend is obese, your odds of also being obese shoot up to 50 to 80 percent. Think about the last time you went out to eat with a group of friends. If you're the only one trying to eat healthy, and everyone else wants burgers and shakes, chances are you end up going where the majority wants to go. Even if there are healthy options available, it's hard to say no when everyone else is getting dessert, and if you don't get your own sugary treat, you might take a couple of bites of theirs.

I am not suggesting that you dump your friends because of their diet, but I am suggesting that you become more aware of the power that people can have over your food choices. Let's review some tips you can implement when navigating social situations around food, so that you can still enjoy being with your friends and also keep on track with your health and nutrition goals. Just because you're avoiding sugar doesn't mean that your social life needs to end—in fact, it can be even better than it already is!

Tips for Managing Social Pressures

TIP 1: Anticipate Potential Temptations

Some triggers are clear and predictable once you look at your situation (flip back to chapter 4 for some examples—snacking-in-front-of-the-TV routines are a perfect example), but some triggering situations are unavoidable. For instance, say your grandmother baked her favorite pie from when she was a kid and wants the whole family to taste it, or your best friend's new baby gender reveal involves cake pops. These situations can make your journey a bit harder to stay on, but a bump in the road doesn't always mean you'll get a flat tire. One taste of a food does not *have* to set you back weeks of progress on your own health journey. But on the same note, you don't have to eat Grandma's pie to show her your love or eat a cake pop to celebrate your friend's new baby. Just because you're breaking up with sugar doesn't mean you shouldn't participate in a festive occasion. If you are able to (and want to) take a bite and walk away, go for it! If not, say you're stuffed from dinner. If they're insistent on your having a piece, offer to take one home with you, and then conveniently forget to ask for it when you're leaving. I like to refer to these types of situations as doing the "politeness dance." Your host is trying to be polite by giving you a treat or making sure you have some to go home with, and you're trying to be polite by obliging them. Nothing wrong with doing this, but don't get tripped by your dance partner. Having situational awareness about what's going to cause you to rebound back to your old self versus not being "rude" and "disrespectful" is completely different!

TIP 2: Come Up with a List of Potential Verbal Responses

Say you're out to lunch with a few coworkers and they want to have dessert with you to "celebrate" a project being complete. While you may no longer be "celebrating" your accomplishments with sweets, you might not necessarily want to preach this to your colleagues. Sometimes, when you feel like you have to explain your reasons not to eat something, it can be awkward, and it's naturally just easier to participate with what the group is doing and eat the darn dessert.

But you don't have to do that. What you eat or drink should have no bearing on what others think of you. And you know that, but in the moment, it can feel awkward to be the person who isn't partici- pating. Why is it that we find it awkward to be the lone wolf and not partake in eating that dessert, or drinking that sugary beverage when with a group? This is a well-known psychological phenom- enon known as "groupthink." Humans naturally want harmony and uniformity among the group and will go along with sometimes irrational or dysfunctional ideas just to be a part of it. Don't let the group sway you to make a poor decision for your health! If you stand out as the dissenter in the group and opt for a non-sugar option, you may just find that others will join you. So, take time out of your day beforehand to form an appropriate response to situ- ations like this, where you may feel peer-pressured to go for the extra treat, to save yourself stress and time in the future. Responses like "I'm already stuffed" or "I'm going to have a coffee instead because I need some energy" can and often do immediately handle things. However, sometimes people are more pressing, so responses like "I'm working on bettering my eating habits" or "I'm being conscious of my water intake, so I don't need a different drink" can be useful when friends and family are aware of your mission to better health. Ideally, it would be great to be able to blurt out "Nah, I'm good" when offered something that you know isn't on your list of things you want to eat or drink. If you can do that, super! You don't need to justify your behavior or food choices to anyone. But the reality is that it isn't always so easy to be that brutally honest (e.g., if you're out with your boss and don't want to come across as rude or ungrateful when they're offering to treat you).

TIP 3: Don't Show Up Without a Plan

When past the point of normal hunger, it's easy to eat the first thing you see, and if that's at a restaurant, it's probably from the bread basket. If you have plans to go out to eat, don't go in blind. Look up the menu prior to going to the restaurant, make a plan, and try your hardest to stick with it. Although some larger chain restaurants post the nutrition information so there's no guesswork involved, not all places do. Before you go, reading the description of the foods on the menu can help you spot hidden sources of sugar and come up with good alternatives. For example, if you want a specific meal but it's loaded with barbecue sauce, you can ask if they'll prepare it with less or no sauce. "On the side" is a common refrain in restaurants these days and no one will judge you, promise. If you know the group you're eating with always splits a couple of appetizers, go in with a low-sugar option and suggest it. If you're not eating out but going to a friend's house instead, bring a low-sugar appetizer so you'll know there'll be something for you to eat. If it's not the venue to bring something, don't make a plate with the first things you see. Look around at the entire table and weigh all your options, then make a plan from there. Although it isn't always possible, try to keep your choices as balanced as possible (having a variety of foods on your plate, not just one or two things, will help you to feel fuller). Once you make your plate, step away from the food and mingle. It's easy to keep picking and eat more than you intended if you're standing next to the hors d'oeuvres table. Lastly, don't be afraid to say no. Sometimes people are food pushers, and whether or not they're trying to sabotage your success, always saying yes can really hinder your goals. Whether you want to share your goals and why you're opting not to have certain foods is completely up to you, but there's nothing wrong with respectfully declining something!

▶•◀

Throughout this chapter, we focused on stress, setbacks, and social pressures, and how they can affect your journey to being sugarless. The biggest takeaway I want you to remember is that you have the power to decide, to do something different for your health and to follow through with it, to stay focused, to cope with stressors and setbacks, and to not be easily swayed by others. By practicing mindfulness, having a great support system, and standing up to social pressures and your environment, this journey won't be stressful—it will be stress-relieving.

You're beginning to become a new person—free from cravings, stress, and most importantly, sugar. I hope you use the tools I've given you to level up your mental well-being and, in turn, reap the physical benefits of eating less sugar—from initial withdrawal symptoms to learning how to cook healthful meals that are free of the harmful addictive ingredient you've been working so hard to get rid of! I hope this next chapter makes you proud of how far you've come . . . and if you haven't started yet, I hope it inspires you just a little bit more to begin your sugarless journey. You have the power and knowledge to take control of your sugar addiction, and you are not alone.

SUGAR-*LESS* FOR LIFE

You may have initially picked up this book because you wanted some advice on how to give up sugar for good. If that sounds familiar, you're obviously not alone. Like so many others, you may have tried to rid your diet of sugar but somehow it would sneak back in, and you'd be hooked all over again. As promised from the beginning, this is not a diet book—it was written to give you the most up-to-date science and psychology on why we eat so much sugar and realistic ways to break your sugar habit once and for all. Hopefully you now feel more empowered than ever to lower the sugar you consume without feeling as if you're on some crazy restrictive diet.

Regardless of which dietary guidelines you refer to, both nationally and globally they stress the same thing: we need to reduce our sugar intake. But people still can't give it up. The most recent recommendation by the World Health Organization (WHO) is to have no more than 10 percent of your calories come from added sugars, and acknowledge that if it were less than 5 percent, it would be even better. Yes, we can argue that people have been starting to decrease their sugar intake over the last decade, but it's not enough. Nationally, most people are still consuming about 13 percent of their calories from sugar. After reading this book, take a sugar inventory of your own typical day and do a quick estimate of how many calories are coming from added sugars—is it 30 percent, 15 percent, closer to 10 percent? It may surprise you. But it doesn't matter where you're starting, it just matters that you are starting! Remember, the goal of this book is to eat less sugar and break the cycle of sugar addiction.

What I want you to walk away with after finishing this book is that after following the plan in *Sugarless*, in due time, maintaining a sugar-less life will become like second nature to you. (If you just chuckled, I don't blame you.) After having tried diet plan after diet plan, you may be at the point where you don't believe *anything* can work. But remember, this isn't a diet; it's a new way of living, and with time, as you grow in confidence around what you want to eat, why you eat it, and re-create your relationship with food, you'll become a new person. A person who is in control and calls the shots. People try to lower their sugar intake all the time—right before the summer, or a big event like a wedding, or if they've received a diagnosis where lowering their sugar would benefit their health. Every New Year's Eve you may say to yourself "no more sugar starting tomorrow," and unfortunately, like most people who set out to make dietary changes for the new year, these changes don't last very long. If it were so easy to eat healthy in our current food environment, it wouldn't be a resolution year after year for so many people. In fact, about 50 percent of people who set out to make dietary changes once January starts report having made the same resolution in the past. Initially, people may beat themselves up over it, but over time, sugar sneaks its way back in and it's just part of their typical diet again.

But that won't be happening to you. You now know about the addictive hold that sugar can have on you, and why willpower is seemingly never enough to curb it. It isn't about willpower—addiction strips us of our will. You now have the skills to change your behaviors and thoughts around food. For many people, it's sometimes easier to throw in the towel. Luckily for you, you now know what to look for. While taking an inventory of what you have available to you at home, what you have stashed away at work, in the car, or wherever you keep food in general, you'll get faster at spotting the sugar on the label. Soon enough you'll be way more label-savvy and you won't need to constantly reference the seemingly endless list of alternative names for sugar. Not only that, but as you start to clear your diet of foods created by companies and start eating real food instead, there will be fewer ingredients to read through on the label. Compare the label of plain oatmeal to an oatmeal breakfast bar. Plain oatmeal has, or should have, one ingredient: oats. Conversely, a popular oat-based breakfast bar (Nature Valley® Soft-Baked Oatmeal Squares) has more than twenty ingredients! It's all about going back to basics. Less is more!

Now you have the knowledge. But, as you now know, having the knowledge about what to do is only half the battle. After reading through chapter 3, you have a good understanding on why even though we know sugar is killing us, it still isn't enough to make us stop consuming it. Our brain is literally addicted to sugar, and breaking that cycle isn't an easy feat. Before you start putting in the actual work to break the cycle of sugar addiction, revisit your quiz results from page 280. Did you take time to process your results? Were you surprised by the results? What did your results tell you about your relationship with food? At that point, you may have felt overwhelmed, upset, or surprised—probably a combo of all three— but you didn't let that stop you. You kept on reading, which shows right there that you WANT to make a change. You could have just put the book down and never looked at it again, but since you're up to the very end of the book, it shows you're motivated and committed to seeing this through. But before starting on the seven steps outlined in chapter 4, don't forget the three ground rules!

Rule 1: There is no rush.

Rule 2: A slipup is not your excuse to give up.

Rule 3: These steps aren't linear.

Always refer to these rules when you feel like it's not going as you would have liked. There will most certainly be times when sugar gets the best of you, but you can't let that completely derail you from all the progress you're making. That's why identifying your trigger foods (and what to have instead) is so important. It is *so* important, in fact, that there's an entire chapter dedicated to it (see chapter 5)! Being more in tune with your body, specifically your hunger and satiety signals, is a skill that takes practice (we can blame all the ultra-processed foods for overriding our satiety signals, making us never feel full despite taking in excessive calories). The good news is, when you revisit your diet and start incorporating real foods with real nutrients, this gets easier. At first it will be a challenge, but remembering your long-term health goals and those three ground rules will make it easier. Research shows that people who stick with their dietary changes longer don't have an "all or nothing" approach; they're flexible and acknowledge that there will be ups and downs. Another tip that was highlighted earlier (as cumbersome as it may seem) is to keep a food diary or any kind of log that works for you. Doing a three-day diary is great, but some people find that sticking with it longer is a helpful way to maintain their success. Writing down what you eat and how you feel can be really eye-opening. You can find patterns between your emotions and the foods you're eating. Further, when you have a better grasp on what you're putting into your body, it's easier to spot where you might be doing great and areas that may benefit from a little help. When considering your food environment and daily routines, it will probably be a struggle at first, but that's where you can use the recipes and tips provided in this book to help! Taking the guesswork out of what you need in the kitchen, what to buy at the grocery store, and other helpful tips to eating less sugar for life are all provided to prevent you from having a setback. Even if you do lapse, you now know not to beat yourself up over it. You have the skills, tools, and power to get back to work, and know that coping with setbacks and not letting a lapse turn into a relapse is crucial. The tips, tricks, recipes, and, most importantly, the scientific facts I've shown you throughout this book will lead you in the future. Now that you're officially armed with the tools to break the sugar addiction, you are more equipped than ever to navigate situations that may have previously derailed you and go sugar-less for life. Just wait until you see the amazing places it takes you!

30 SUGAR-*LESS* RECIPES

If you find yourself uncomfortable in the kitchen, you aren't alone! Many people struggle to figure out what to make, how to make it, when to make it, and how to keep it healthy. As humans, we can become indecisive and jumbled in our food choices as we juggle our hectic lives. Healthy eating does not need to be a daunting task. It can be made simple, and it's an easy way to control what goes into our bodies. Many prepared foods from a grocery store or restaurant are *full* of unnecessary added sugars. Eating these foods in excess can increase your chances of developing chronic disease, so why not take control of your meals in your own kitchen? Your health should be a priority, so let's get into the kitchen and make some meals that will give your body what it needs and help it feel good.

The recipes here have been specifically designed to help you beat your addiction to sugar. The ingredients have been carefully curated, and I've tested the recipes to ensure that the foods not only taste yummy, but will keep you full longer and manage your sugar cravings. I have also designed them to be versatile, so you can adapt them to include ingredients that you prefer. After a little experimentation in the kitchen, these recipes will become delicious staples in your sugarless life.

Quick Cooking Tips

Before you dig into the recipes, here are some quick tips that can make your food prep easier.

- Grocery shop for a week's worth of eating. You will be less likely to grab convenience foods when you know you are stocked up at home.

- Keep your pantry well stocked with dry good staples so you always have options.

- Precook your grains the day before, if time permits.

- Cut the time of cooking vegetables in half by first precooking them in the microwave.

- Take some time in the morning to assemble your recipe ingredients for dinner. Need to chop a few vegetables? Go ahead and chop them up, then place them in a container in the fridge so they are ready to go when it's time to make dinner. Or do this over the weekend with the vegetables you need for several meals that you plan to create during the week.

- Find all the recipes you want to make for the upcoming week. Using the ingredients lists from those recipes, make a grocery list so you know what you need to buy and what is on hand at your home.

- Keep a running grocery list easily accessible. Run out of milk? Write it down so you don't forget to buy more.

- Cook in batches and freeze leftovers. If there is a particular recipe you really like, double it and keep one batch in the freezer to use if you run out of ideas for a meal later on, or if you get lazy and don't feel like cooking!

- Give your leftovers new life. The grilled chicken you make tonight can become chicken tacos tomorrow.

- If it makes sense, keep a compost bowl nearby when prepping your ingredients so you can keep your workspace clean. If you have a composter at home, feed it your scraps after you are done prepping your meals! If you have a garden, kitchen compost is a great way to return nutrients to the soil. If you are new to composting, note that composting cooked food isn't recommended.

- Clean as you go. Don't let every dirty dish and utensil pile up so they're all waiting for you at the end! This makes cooking cumbersome—cleaning little by little as you prep helps make things more manageable.

Tools of the Trade

You don't need a million gadgets to be a good cook, but there are some items that can make meal prep easier. Here are my suggestions for items to have on hand to make cooking a breeze.

1. Chef's knife
2. Paring knife
3. Cutting boards
4. Can opener
5. Measuring cups/spoons
6. Mixing bowls
7. Colander
8. Vegetable peeler
9. Whisk
10. Grater
11. Kitchen shears (scissors)
12. Stainless-steel skillet
13. Sauté pan
14. Saucepan
15. Large pot
16. Baking sheet
17. Casserole dish
18. Blender (immersion blender or standing blender)
19. Stirring spoons
20. Spatula
21. Tongs
22. Ladle
23. Oven mitts
24. Instant-read thermometer
25. Airtight food storage containers

Kitchen Staples

It helps to have some items on hand when prepping meals. These items are used in many of my recipes and are staples with long shelf lives. They are essential for any well-stocked kitchen, especially a sugarless one.

OILS AND VINEGARS: Extra-virgin olive oil, canola oil, toasted sesame oil, avocado oil, red wine vinegar, distilled white vinegar, apple cider vinegar, rice vinegar, white wine vinegar

CANS AND JARS: Tomato products (diced tomatoes, tomato sauce, tomato paste—make sure there's no added sugar); low-sodium broth (chicken, beef, vegetable); tuna, chicken; low-sodium beans and chickpeas

GRAINS AND STARCHES: Rice, quinoa, pasta (one long shape, one short, and one chunky), plain bread crumbs, crackers, dried lentils

NUTS/NUT BUTTERS: Almonds, walnuts, almond butter, cashew butter, peanut butter (again, check the labels and make sure there is no added sugar)

PRODUCE: Garlic, onions, potatoes, lemons, limes (these tend to last longer; you can get other produce you plan to use up right away when you do your weekly shopping)

POULTRY AND DAIRY: Eggs, unsalted butter, cheese, milk

CONDIMENTS AND SAUCES: Mustard (yellow and Dijon), mayonnaise, salsa, hot sauce, low-sodium soy sauce

BAKING: All-purpose flour, cornmeal, rolled oats, cornstarch, baking soda, baking powder, pure vanilla extract, bittersweet baking chocolate, dried fruit, raw cacao powder

Recipes

Breakfast

- Blender Pancakes with Maple Sauce (p. 216)
- Sugarless Granola (p. 218)
- Waffles and Cream (p. 219)
- Eggy Roasted Red Pepper Breakfast Wraps (p. 221)
- Oatmeal Breakfast Cookies (p. 223)

Lunch or Dinner

- Mini Burger Bite Skewers (p. 224)
- Creamy Tomato and Roasted Red Pepper Soup with Grilled Halloumi (p. 226)
- Coconut Avocado Lime Soup (p. 228)
- Pulled Chicken Burrito Bowl (p. 230)
- Baked Salmon Sushi Rolls with Cilantro-Lime Rice (p. 232)
- Chickpea-Avocado Sandwich (p. 235)
- Stuffed Avocados (p. 237)
- BLT Egg Salad Lettuce Cups (p. 239)

Side Dishes

- Cold Sesame Rice Noodle Salad (p. 240)

- Rainbow Salad with Lemon-Herb Vinaigrette (p. 242)

- No-Fry Teriyaki-Pineapple Rice (p. 244)

- Old Bay® Roasted Crispy Chickpeas (p. 246)

- Sheet Pan Roasted Root Veggies (p. 247)

Condiments

- Sugarless Coffee Creamer (p. 249)

- Sugarless BBQ Sauce (p. 250)

- Sugarless Creamy Caesar Dressing (p. 252)

- Sugarless Ranch Dip (p. 253)

- Sugarless Classic Ketchup (p. 254)

Desserts and Snacks

- Strawberry Shortcake Parfait (p. 255)

- Frozen Yogurt Bark with Nuts and Berries (p. 257)

- Salted Caramel-ish Rice Puff Bars (p. 258)

- Blueberry Oatmeal Muffins (p. 260)

- Whole-Fruit Frozen Rocket Pops (p. 262)

- Unbelievable Ice Cream Sundae (p. 264)

- Easy Flaxseed Crackers with Olive Hummus (p. 266)

Blender Pancakes with Maple Sauce

Makes 6 large pancakes

My favorite memory from childhood is of my mom making pancakes on Saturday morning while I watched cartoons! Here I have re-created that childhood favorite without the added sugar. Blender pancakes are an easy way to keep your kitchen clean and satisfy the whole family. By replacing traditional maple syrup with a homemade maple sauce, you can avoid many grams of added sugar.

INGREDIENTS

For the pancakes

½ cup unsweetened applesauce

1 cup milk of choice (see Note)

3 tablespoons unsalted butter, melted

1½ cups all-purpose flour

2 teaspoons baking powder

1 teaspoon ground cinnamon

¼ teaspoon fine sea salt

Nonstick spray

For the maple sauce

½ cup unsweetened applesauce

1 tablespoon maple extract, or more to taste

MAKE THE PANCAKES: In your blender, combine the applesauce, milk, melted butter, flour, baking powder, cinnamon, and salt. Blend on high until smooth, 45 to 60 seconds, stopping to scrape down the sides as needed.

Heat a large skillet over medium heat and coat with nonstick spray. Pour ¾ cup of the pancake batter onto the pan for each pancake. Cook for 2 to 5 minutes per side, flipping once when bubbles form along the edge and surface of each pancake. Transfer the pancakes to a plate and repeat with the remaining batter.

JUST BEFORE SERVING, MAKE THE MAPLE SAUCE: Rinse out your blender. Combine the applesauce, maple extract, and 1 tablespoon water in the clean blender and blend on high until smooth, about 30 seconds.

To serve, plate your pancakes and pour the maple sauce on top or serve it alongside.

Store the pancakes and maple sauce in separate airtight containers in the refrigerator for up to 4 days.

Notes: Plain pancakes seem boring? While the batter is cooking, a few minutes before flipping, add banana slices, fresh berries, or 100 percent cacao dark chocolate chips! These pancakes can be changed up in many ways to make them unique each and every time you cook them for breakfast.

Instead of regular milk, you can use an unsweetened nondairy milk like oat milk.

Sugarless Granola

Makes 3 cups

Granola is a great topping on smoothie bowls, pudding, yogurt, and oatmeal. It is also delicious alone. This recipe has sweetness from the dried currants, which pairs perfectly with a touch of saltiness and nutty flavor from the cashews and almond butter.

INGREDIENTS

2 cups rolled oats

¼ cup raw cashews, chopped

¼ cup dried currants or other dried fruit

2 tablespoons unsweetened coconut flakes

1 tablespoon chia seeds

1 tablespoon sesame seeds

½ teaspoon ground cinnamon

½ teaspoon fine sea salt

⅓ cup unsweetened almond butter

Preheat the oven to 325°F. Line a small baking sheet or a 9 by 13-inch baking dish with parchment paper.

In a medium bowl, combine the oats, cashews, currants, coconut, chia seeds, sesame seeds, cinnamon, and salt. Fold in the almond butter. Spread the mixture evenly over the prepared baking sheet.

Bake for 10 minutes, then remove the pan from the oven, stir the granola, and spread it evenly again. Bake for 5 minutes more, or until golden brown. Cool completely before serving or storing.

Store in an airtight container at room temperature for up to 1 week.

Notes: Any type of nut butter will work in this recipe.

Keep an eye on the currants and coconut to make sure they do not burn.

Waffles and Cream

Makes 8 waffles

Waffles are my go-to when my family wants something yummy and comforting but we are short on prep time. This modern take on an old-fashioned breakfast treat allows you to indulge a little without the added sugar. These energy-dense waffles are topped with a simple whipped cream paired with nutritious cacao nibs or fruit. You might just forget this is breakfast and think you are having dessert!

INGREDIENTS

For the waffles

2 cups all-purpose flour or whole-wheat flour

1 tablespoon baking powder

½ teaspoon fine sea salt

2 large eggs

1 cup milk of choice

1 teaspoon pure vanilla extract

½ cup (1 stick) unsalted butter, melted

Canola oil spray, for greasing the waffle iron

For the topping

½ cup heavy cream

½ teaspoon pure vanilla extract

¼ cup cacao nibs (optional)

Fruit of choice (optional)

RECIPE CONTINUES

MAKE THE WAFFLES: Preheat a waffle iron to medium.

In a large bowl, combine the flour, baking powder, and salt. In medium bowl, combine the eggs, milk, and vanilla. Add the wet ingredients to the dry ingredients and stir a few times to combine. Add the melted butter and stir to incorporate. You don't want to overmix the batter.

Spray the waffle iron lightly with canola oil. Add approximately 3 tablespoons of the batter to the middle of the iron and cook according to the manufacturer's instructions until the edges are golden and the waffle is cooked through, 2 to 3 minutes. Transfer the cooked waffle to a plate and repeat with the remaining batter.

MAKE THE TOPPING: Whisk the cream and vanilla in a small bowl until stiff peaks form, 2 to 3 minutes.

To serve, divide the waffles among four plates, add a spoonful of the cream on top of the waffles, and finish with a sprinkling of cacao nibs and/or fruit.

Store leftover waffles in an airtight container in the refrigerator for 3 to 5 days or in the freezer for up to 4 months. When reheating from the freezer, just pop the frozen waffles into the toaster. The whipped topping can also be stored in an airtight container in the refrigerator for up to 3 days, but it tastes better fresh.

Note: Cacao nibs are a great sugarless alternative to chocolate sprinkles. But what are they? Chocolate comes from cacao beans, and cacao nibs are simply crushed-up bits of meat from the raw beans. You can enjoy a dark chocolaty taste with the nutritional benefits of cacao, like heart-healthy flavonoids and antioxidants, without all the processing and added sugar that you get when eating chocolate.

Eggy Roasted Red Pepper Breakfast Wraps

Serves 4

This is my favorite breakfast to prep in bulk on the weekend, because it can last my family all week. A protein-packed breakfast not only keeps us fuller for longer, it also helps balance our blood sugar levels in the morning. Eggs are a versatile way to get protein into your day—especially if you don't like meat! By prepping batches of these wraps and storing them in freezer bags, you can have quick breakfasts that are easy to prepare and healthy throughout the week.

INGREDIENTS

1 cup plain Greek yogurt

½ cup roasted red peppers

1 tablespoon spicy brown mustard

1 teaspoon fine sea salt

1 teaspoon freshly ground black pepper

1 teaspoon garlic powder

4 hard-boiled large eggs, peeled and chopped

½ cup cherry tomatoes, halved

½ cup artichoke hearts, diced

Arugula

4 large whole-wheat tortillas

In a food processor, combine the yogurt, red peppers, mustard, salt, black pepper, and garlic powder. Pulse until the mixture is smooth, about 1 minute. Set the sauce aside in a small bowl.

RECIPE CONTINUES

In a large bowl, combine the chopped eggs, tomatoes, artichoke hearts, and arugula. Gently toss to combine, then add the sauce and toss again until well combined.

To assemble the wraps, lay out the tortillas on your work surface. Scoop ½ cup of the egg mixture into the center of each wrap. Working with one at a time, fold the top of tortilla over the filling, then tuck in the sides and continue rolling toward yourself, creating a tightly packed wrap!

You may store the preassembled wraps in an airtight container in the refrigerator for up to 3 days or in a freezer bag in the freezer for up to 1 month. Take frozen wraps out of the freezer and defrost in the refrigerator overnight before eating.

Note: Not a huge red pepper fan? Try swapping them out for sun-dried tomatoes! With no sugar and concentrated flavor, sun-dried tomatoes and roasted red peppers are both great ways to add flavor to a dish.

Oatmeal Breakfast Cookies

Makes 6 cookies

Tired of boring old regular oatmeal? Sick of overnight oats? To change things up, try turning your breakfast oatmeal into cookies! This recipe pairs fiber-rich oats with fruit for sweetness. These oatmeal breakfast cookies are great for digestion and make the perfect recipe to wake up to.

INGREDIENTS

    1 ripe medium banana

    1½ cups rolled oats

    1 teaspoon baking powder

    ¼ teaspoon pure vanilla extract

    ¼ teaspoon fine sea salt

Preheat the oven to 350°F. Line a baking sheet with parchment paper.

In a medium bowl, thoroughly mash the banana using a fork. Add the oats, baking powder, vanilla, and salt. Stir until well combined. Form the mixture into 6 even balls and place them on the prepared baking sheet, then press down on each one with your palm to form rounds approximately ¼ inch think. (The cookies will not spread during baking.)

Bake for about 15 minutes, until the cookies start to turn golden brown. Let cool for 10 minutes before serving or storing.

Store in an airtight container lined with a paper towel (to absorb any moisture) in the refrigerator for 2 to 3 days.

Note: The unbaked cookies can even be frozen to bake later! After you've formed the dough into rounds, store them in a freezer-safe container with parchment paper between each layer, then bake from frozen.

Mini Burger Bite Skewers

Makes 14 skewers

These burger bite skewers are my go-to dinner during the week. You can even double the recipe and serve them as an appetizer at any get-together.

INGREDIENTS

For the burger bites

1 large egg

1 tablespoon chopped fresh basil

1 tablespoon chopped fresh parsley

1 teaspoon garlic powder

1 teaspoon onion powder

½ teaspoon fine sea salt

½ teaspoon freshly ground black pepper

1 pound ground beef (80% lean)

¼ cup bread crumbs

1 tablespoon extra-virgin olive oil

For the skewers

7 cherry tomatoes, halved

¼ head romaine or iceberg lettuce, torn into small pieces

14 pickle slices

14 (½-inch) cubes cheddar cheese (from an 8-ounce block)

Sugarless Classic Ketchup (p. 254), for serving

MAKE THE BURGER BITES: Beat the egg in a large bowl. Whisk in the basil, parsley, garlic powder, onion powder, salt, and pepper. Add the ground beef and bread crumbs and mix with clean hands, or a spoon, until fully combined. Form the meat mixture into fourteen 1½-inch balls.

In a large skillet, heat the olive oil over medium heat. When the oil is shimmering, add the burger bites. Cook, rotating the burger bites to brown on all sides, until cooked through, 12 to 15 minutes.

ASSEMBLE THE SKEWERS: Slide each cooked burger bite onto a 4-inch-long mini skewer. Add half a cherry tomato, slice of lettuce, pickle slice, and cube of cheese to each skewer.

Serve the burger bite skewers with sugar-free ketchup alongside.

Store the skewers in an airtight container in the refrigerator for up to 3 days.

Note: These can also be grilled, if you want! Just form the meat mixture into balls, then spear them on heat-safe skewers and cook them either on an outdoor barbecue or a grill pan on the stove, cooking as directed.

Creamy Tomato and Roasted Red Pepper Soup with Grilled Halloumi

Serves 4

If I had to pick my last meal, it would be a grilled cheese sandwich. Nothing feels as warm and nostalgic to me as that gooey melted cheese and crisp toast. Comfort food can be healthy, too! This take on your favorite cold-weather dish is sweetened naturally with roasted red peppers, and the grilled halloumi cheese is lower in carbohydrates than a traditional grilled cheese sandwich.

INGREDIENTS

1 tablespoon extra-virgin olive oil

1 cup diced white onion (1 small)

1 medium carrot, shredded

½ teaspoon fine sea salt

2 garlic cloves, minced

3 tablespoons tomato paste

1 (14-ounce) can diced tomatoes, drained

1 (12-ounce) jar roasted red peppers, drained

1 cup vegetable broth

½ teaspoon dried thyme

Freshly ground black pepper

1 cup milk of choice

8 ounces halloumi cheese, cut into 4 (¼-inch-thick) slices

In a Dutch oven, heat the olive oil over medium-high heat. When the oil is shimmering, add the onion and carrot, and sauté until the onion starts to become translucent, about 5 minutes. Reduce the heat to medium and add the salt, garlic, and tomato paste. Cook for 1 minute, stirring occasionally. Add the diced tomatoes, red peppers, broth, thyme, and black pepper to taste. Reduce the heat to low and cook, stirring occasionally, for about 20 minutes, until thickened.

Carefully transfer the mixture to a blender and pulse until smooth, about 1 minute (or use an immersion blender directly in the pot). Return the mixture to the pot and stir in the milk. Cook over low heat for 1 to 2 minutes, until warmed through.

Meanwhile, heat a grill pan or nonstick skillet over medium heat. Add the sliced cheese to the pan and cook for 3 to 4 minutes, then flip and cook for 2 minutes on the second side.

Divide the soup among four bowls and serve immediately with the grilled halloumi alongside.

Store leftover soup and halloumi in separate airtight containers in the refrigerator for 3 to 5 days.

Coconut Avocado Lime Soup

Serves 4

I love to have soups on hand in the fridge or freezer for a quick meal. It may come as a shock that this soup is served cold, but the flavors stand out this way. The healthy fats from the coconut milk and avocado are perfectly balanced with the fresh lime juice and salt, and will help you feel fuller, longer.

INGREDIENTS

1 large head cauliflower, chopped into 1-inch florets

2 ripe avocados, pitted, peeled, and chilled

½ cup vegetable broth, chilled

1 cup canned unsweetened coconut milk, full-fat

Juice of 1 lime

2 tablespoons chopped fresh cilantro, plus more for garnish

1 garlic clove, peeled

¼ teaspoon fine sea salt

¼ teaspoon freshly ground black pepper

⅛ teaspoon red pepper flakes (optional)

In a medium pot, combine the cauliflower and ¼ cup water. Bring the water to a simmer over medium-low heat, then cover with a lid. Steam the cauliflower, stirring occasionally with a rubber spatula to ensure it doesn't burn, for about 10 minutes, until tender. Remove the pot from the heat.

Drain the cauliflower and transfer it to a blender. Add the avocados, broth, coconut milk, lime juice, cilantro, garlic, salt, black pepper, and red pepper flakes. Blend for 30 seconds, or until fully combined and smooth. Refrigerate for at least 20 minutes and up to 1 hour before serving.

To serve, pour the soup into bowls and garnish with fresh cilantro.

Store the soup in an airtight container in the refrigerator for up to 5 days or in the freezer for up to 6 months. Defrost frozen soup in the refrigerator before serving. Serve cold or at room temperature.

Notes: Be sure the avocados are perfectly ripe. They should be soft and easy to cut into, but not brown. This will ensure that the soup is fresh and flavorful.

If you do not want to steam the cauliflower on the stovetop, you can buy a bag of frozen cauliflower and steam it in the microwave.

Pulled Chicken Burrito Bowl

Serves 4

If someone asked me to choose my favorite Mexican dish, it would be a burrito bowl. This burrito bowl can be a nutritious dinner or lunch. Pinto beans are an excellent source of fiber, the perfect addition to a meal to keep your blood sugar from spiking. Nutritious nonstarchy vegetables such as tomatoes and cucumbers support healthy blood sugar levels and can help you avoid cravings.

INGREDIENTS

1 pound boneless, skinless chicken breasts (about 2 large)

2 tablespoons extra-virgin olive oil

1 (1-ounce) packet taco seasoning

1 avocado, pitted and peeled

½ medium red onion, finely diced

Juice of ½ lime

Fine sea salt

2 cups cooked brown rice

1½ cups cherry tomatoes, quartered

1 cup salsa

½ cup diced cucumber

¼ cup plain low-fat Greek yogurt

1 (15.5-ounce) can pinto beans, drained and rinsed

Preheat the oven to 325°F. Line a rimmed baking sheet with parchment paper.

In a large bowl, combine the chicken, olive oil, and taco seasoning. Coat the chicken evenly in the oil and seasoning.

Transfer the chicken to the prepared baking sheet. Bake for about 30 minutes, until golden brown and cooked through. Let the chicken rest for 10 minutes, then shred with two forks.

While the chicken cooks, use a fork to mash the avocado in a small bowl. Stir in the onion and lime juice and season the guacamole with salt to taste.

To serve, spoon ½ cup of the rice into each bowl. Divide the cooked chicken, tomatoes, salsa, cucumber, guacamole, yogurt, and beans among the bowls.

Store unused portions of the ingredients in separate airtight containers in the refrigerator for up to 4 days. When preparing leftovers, heat the rice and chicken separately, then top with the cold ingredients.

Note: Can't find pinto beans in the grocery store? Black beans or navy beans make a great substitute! They contain similar amounts of fiber and are a great plant-based protein source. And if you are out of your favorite salsa, have no fear—you can replace the salsa with sugar-free hot sauce, or put together a quick homemade salsa with chopped tomatoes, jalapeño, cilantro, and onion.

Baked Salmon Sushi Rolls with Cilantro-Lime Rice

Serves 2

Sugar in your sushi? You bet there is! Many sushi rolls have added sugar because of the sauces that are used when mixing up the ingredients. But you can easily make your own sugarless rolls at home! It might take some practice to get used to rolling sushi rolls, but that is what makes this a fun recipe. This savory dish is packed with fresh flavors from the lemon juice, parsley, and avocado. The cilantro-lime rice is just as much a star as the baked salmon, and they pair perfectly together. This can be easily be turned into a dinner bowl—just arrange the rice, salmon, avocado, and crushed seaweed sheets in a bowl and serve!

INGREDIENTS

For the cilantro-lime rice

1 cup long-grain white rice

1 tablespoon extra-virgin olive oil

½ teaspoon fine sea salt

Zest and juice of 1 lime

1 garlic clove, minced

¼ cup chopped fresh cilantro

For the baked salmon

1 (6-ounce) salmon fillet

Juice of 1 small lemon

2 tablespoons chopped fresh parsley

½ teaspoon garlic powder

½ teaspoon onion powder

¼ teaspoon fine sea salt

For the sushi rolls

2 nori seaweed sheets

1 avocado, pitted, peeled, and thinly sliced

1 tablespoon toasted sesame seeds

Preheat the oven to 450°F. Line a small baking sheet with parchment paper.

MAKE THE CILANTRO-LIME RICE: In a large saucepan, bring 2 cups water to a boil over high heat. Add the rice, olive oil, and salt. Cover, reduce the heat to low, and simmer for 15 to 20 minutes, until the rice is soft and fluffy. Remove from the heat and stir in the lime zest, lime juice, garlic, and cilantro. Set aside until cool enough to handle.

WHILE THE RICE IS COOKING, MAKE THE SALMON: Place the salmon skin side down on the prepared pan. Season with the lemon juice, parsley, garlic powder, onion powder, and salt. Rub the seasonings over the salmon to ensure it is evenly coated. Bake for 12 to 15 minutes, until cooked through. Set aside until cool enough to handle.

ASSEMBLE THE SUSHI ROLLS: Lay out a nori sheet on top of a bamboo rolling mat with the rough side of the sheet facing up. Add about half the cilantro-lime rice and evenly spread it out over the nori, leaving ½-inch border at the top and bottom edges. Place thin slices of the avocado in the middle of the rice. Cut the salmon fillet in half lengthwise and lay one piece next to the avocado. Sprinkle with

RECIPE CONTINUES

half the sesame seeds and, using the bamboo mat, begin to roll up the nori and filling. Slice the sushi roll crosswise into 8 equal pieces. Repeat with the remaining ingredients to make a second roll. Serve immediately.

Store the sushi rolls in an airtight container in the refrigerator for 1 to 2 days, but eat them as soon as possible for peak freshness.

Notes: Nori seaweed sheets are best for durability and rolling. If you don't have a bamboo rolling mat, plastic wrap or a tea cloth can be used to roll the sushi. Also, note that these rolls are pretty fat! If you want a tighter roll, you can use half the amount of rice called for and reduce the salmon to 4 ounces.

Chickpea-Avocado Sandwich

Makes 2 sandwiches

My two favorite foods—chickpeas and avocados—get married in this dish. The combination of chickpea and avocado gives you a filling, high-protein sandwich. It requires no baking or cooking (although I do recommend toasting the bread to add the perfect bite!), and can be made within 10 minutes.

INGREDIENTS

For the filling

> 1 cup canned chickpeas, drained and rinsed
>
> 1 avocado, pitted and peeled
>
> 1 celery stalk, chopped (about 3 tablespoons)
>
> ¼ small cucumber, chopped (about 2 tablespoons)
>
> 2 tablespoons chopped fresh cilantro
>
> 1 tablespoon fresh lemon juice
>
> ¼ teaspoon garlic powder
>
> ¼ teaspoon onion powder
>
> ¼ teaspoon fine sea salt

For the sandwiches

> 4 slices whole-wheat bread, toasted if desired
>
> 4 tomato slices
>
> 2 large lettuce leaves
>
> Sugarless Ranch Dip (see p. 253), for dipping (optional)

MAKE THE FILLING: In a medium bowl, combine the chickpeas, avocado, celery, cucumber, cilantro, lemon juice, garlic powder, onion powder, and salt. Using a potato masher or fork, press the chickpeas until they are mashed and all the ingredients are combined.

MAKE THE SANDWICHES: Take one slice of bread and top it with a slice of tomato, then a piece of lettuce, then half the chickpea-avocado filling, then another slice of tomato, and finally top with a second slice of bread. Repeat to assemble a second sandwich.

Slice the sandwiches in half and serve with ranch alongside for dipping, if you like.

Store the chickpea-avocado filling in an airtight container in the refrigerator for 1 to 2 days. The avocado will start to brown after 1 day, so I recommend eating it as soon as possible.

Note: For a smoother texture and added creaminess, you can remove the skins from the chickpeas. To do this, roll the chickpeas around gently on a clean tea cloth or shake them in a colander to separate them. Otherwise, the skins will remain whole when you mash the chickpeas, resulting in a chunkier-textured mixture.

Stuffed Avocados

Serves 4

These stuffed avocados will keep you feeling full and satisfied! You only need 20 minutes to whip this up, and the flavors work great together. This recipe has many flexible ingredients, so you can substitute any of your favorite vegetables for the zucchini and bell pepper. Plus, there is no bowl required for serving, since the avocado skins hold all the ingredients. All you need is a spoon!

INGREDIENTS

1 tablespoon extra-virgin olive oil

¼ cup diced zucchini

¼ cup diced bell pepper (any color)

1 garlic clove, minced

2 tablespoons minced white onion

¼ cup shredded cooked chicken

¼ cup cooked white rice

1 tablespoon fresh lime juice, plus more for serving

1 teaspoon chopped fresh cilantro or parsley,
    plus more for serving

¼ teaspoon fine sea salt

¼ teaspoon freshly ground black pepper

2 ripe avocados

In a saucepan, heat the olive oil over medium heat. Add the zucchini, bell pepper, garlic, and onion and cook, stirring occasionally, for 15 minutes, or until softened. Remove from the heat and transfer the mixture to a bowl. Add the chicken, rice, lime juice, cilantro, salt, and black pepper and mix gently to combine.

RECIPE CONTINUES

To serve, cut the avocados in half and discard the pits, but keep the skins on. Add a rounded ¼ cup of the filling to the center of each avocado half. Garnish with a squeeze of lime juice and some cilantro.

The filling will stay fresh in an airtight container in the refrigerator for 2 to 3 days. Halve, pit, and fill the avocados right before serving so the flesh is fresh and green.

Notes: To prevent browning of the avocado flesh, squeeze lime juice over the cut surfaces after halving the avocados.

These are great served with a cold avocado and warm filling. You can use rotisserie or leftover cooked chicken for this dish, or replace the chicken with any type of protein. Alternatives I recommend include chopped hard-boiled eggs, flaked salmon, and cubed tofu.

BLT Egg Salad Lettuce Cups

Makes 4 servings

One of the best ways to curb cravings is to eat foods that keep you feeling full longer, and that means getting more protein in your meals. Unlike the traditional BLT, which has little protein, this fresh and tasty version adds protein-rich eggs to the mix. This dish may become your go-to for lunch or a quick dinner at home.

INGREDIENTS

6 hard-boiled large eggs, peeled and chopped

½ cup diced tomato (1 small)

⅓ cup mayonnaise

¼ cup diced celery (from 2 stalks)

2 tablespoons diced red onion

1 teaspoon Dijon mustard

Fine sea salt and freshly ground black pepper

8 butter lettuce leaves

3 slices no-sugar-added bacon, cooked until crisp and then chopped, or ⅓ cup bacon bits

In a medium bowl, combine the eggs, tomato, mayonnaise, celery, onion, and mustard. Taste and season with salt and pepper. Cover and refrigerate for at least 30 minutes and up to 1 hour before serving.

To serve, top each lettuce leaf with a heaping ¼ cup of the egg salad and finish with a sprinkling of bacon.

This salad doesn't store well, so enjoy it right away.

Cold Sesame Rice Noodle Salad

Serves 2

When I am busy or tired, sometimes the last thing I want to do is cook, so simple recipes are essential. This one falls into that category. It is light and refreshing—plus, it keeps fresh for days in the fridge. Make a large bowl of noodle salad, and you probably won't be able to put the fork down. The flavors build as you eat it.

INGREDIENTS

For the dressing

¼ cup coconut aminos or low-sodium soy sauce

1 tablespoon rice vinegar

1 tablespoon toasted sesame oil

1 teaspoon chopped fresh cilantro or parsley, plus more
   for garnish

¼ teaspoon red pepper flakes

Pinch of fine sea salt

For the noodle salad

1 ounce rice noodles

1 large carrot (about 10 ounces)

1 medium cucumber (about 10 ounces), peeled

MAKE THE DRESSING: In a large bowl, combine the coconut aminos, vinegar, sesame oil, cilantro, red pepper flakes, and salt.

MAKE THE NOODLE SALAD: Cook the rice noodles according to the package directions. Drain well and set aside to cool.

Using a vegetable peeler or spiralizer, cut the carrot and cucumber into thin "noodles." Add the vegetable noodles and cooked rice noodles to the bowl with the dressing and toss to combine. Serve immediately.

The dressing and noodles can be stored in separate airtight containers for 3 to 5 days. Mix just before serving.

Note: Try some other additions in this salad, like fresh mint or mango for added sweetness. If you want to include some additional protein, add leftover chicken or tofu.

Rainbow Salad with Lemon-Herb Vinaigrette

Serves 4

Salads can go from healthy to sugar bomb in an instant when you add most store-bought dressings and toppings like candied nuts. This simple salad and sugarless dressing will become your go-to for eating the rainbow! It packs so many colorful and nutrient-dense ingredients into one bowl and is paired with a savory vinaigrette that you can prepare on its own and keep handy for serving with other green salads. For some extra protein, top with crispy tofu or grilled chicken.

INGREDIENTS

For the salad

3 cups coarsely chopped stemmed kale leaves (from 1 bunch)

1 cup shredded romaine or iceberg lettuce (½ small head)

¼ cup shredded purple cabbage (¼ small head)

1 large carrot, sliced into coins

1 large cucumber, peeled and sliced into rounds

½ cup cherry tomatoes, halved

1 cup cooked quinoa, cooled

For the dressing

½ cup extra-virgin olive oil

¼ cup fresh lemon juice

2 tablespoons spicy brown mustard

¼ teaspoon dried oregano

¼ teaspoon dried basil

¼ teaspoon garlic powder

¼ teaspoon fine sea salt

¼ teaspoon freshly ground black pepper

MAKE THE SALAD: In a large bowl, toss together the kale, lettuce, cabbage, carrot, cucumber, tomatoes, and quinoa.

MAKE THE DRESSING: In a container with a lid (mason jars with screw-top lids work well here), combine the olive oil, lemon juice, mustard, oregano, basil, garlic powder, salt, and pepper. Cover and shake until fully combined, about 10 seconds.

ASSEMBLE THE SALAD: When ready to serve, pour the dressing over the salad and mix well.

Store the salad in an airtight container in the fridge for 2 to 3 days. Store the dressing in a sealed jar or container in the refrigerator for up to 1 week. Add the dressing to the salad just before serving to prevent the lettuce from becoming soggy.

Notes: When stored in the fridge, the oil will solidify. It will return to its liquid state after 10 minutes on the counter. For a more tender texture, massage the kale by squeezing it in your hands for 1 to 2 minutes to soften it. You can add 1 tablespoon olive oil and a dash of salt before massaging to make it soften more quickly, but this is optional.

This recipe is also very versatile in terms of the green you can use. Other greens that work well are arugula, spinach, and spring mix.

No-Fry Teriyaki-Pineapple Rice

Serves 2

Asian fried rice dishes are delicious, but they often have added sugar. This dish combines the flavors you love from fried rice with a healthier twist. It is a great addition to your plate next to any protein and vegetables for lunch or dinner. Not only is it rich in flavor, the pineapple also adds the perfect touch of sweetness.

INGREDIENTS

For the rice

1 cup long-grain white rice

½ cup diced pineapple

½ cup chopped carrots

¼ cup chopped scallions

½ teaspoon fine sea salt

For the teriyaki sauce

1 teaspoon cornstarch

½ cup low-sodium soy sauce

½ teaspoon onion powder

½ teaspoon garlic powder

¼ teaspoon red pepper flakes

¼ teaspoon ground ginger

MAKE THE RICE: In a large saucepan, bring 2 cups water to a boil over high heat. Add the rice. Cover and reduce the heat to low. Simmer for 15 to 20 minutes, until the rice is soft and fluffy. While the rice is cooking, prepare the teriyaki sauce.

MAKE THE TERIYAKI SAUCE: In a small saucepan, whisk together the cornstarch and 1 teaspoon water over low heat until combined. Whisk in the soy sauce, onion powder, garlic powder, red pepper flakes, and ginger. Allow it to simmer for 5 minutes, or until thickened.

ASSEMBLE THE TERIYAKI-PINEAPPLE RICE: Once the rice has finished cooking, stir in the pineapple, carrots, scallions, and salt.

Pour the teriyaki sauce over the rice and mix until combined. Serve immediately.

Store the rice in an airtight container in the refrigerator for up to 5 days. If you make the teriyaki sauce separately, it will stay fresh in an airtight container in the refrigerator for up to 2 weeks.

Notes: The teriyaki sauce is very flavorful. If you want to add protein such as chicken or tofu to this recipe, I would recommend marinating it in the teriyaki sauce for 30 minutes, then cooking it with the sauce for bold flavor.

The carrots and scallions are just two options here—feel free to add any vegetables or fresh herbs you have available. You can use canned pineapple or fresh pineapple; just make sure there is no added sugar if it's canned.

Old Bay® Roasted Crispy Chickpeas

Serves 2

I originally created this recipe for my teenage daughter. It started as a healthy snack that I could pack in her lunch, but it soon became a family favorite, and now we make it once a week, at least. Chickpeas are a great source of protein and fiber, the two main things you want to look for in a healthy snack. The protein will keep you feeling full, while the fiber is good for optimizing your blood sugar levels, which can help with sugar cravings. This spicy snack is great between meals, or even as a side dish for your dinner.

INGREDIENTS

1 (15.5-ounce) can chickpeas, drained and rinsed

1 tablespoon extra-virgin olive oil

1 tablespoon Old Bay® Seasoning

Preheat the oven to 325°F. Line a rimmed baking sheet with aluminum foil.

Put the chickpeas in a medium bowl. Add the olive oil and toss to coat the chickpeas. Add the Old Bay® and toss again to coat.

Pour the chickpeas over the prepared baking sheet, spreading them into an even layer. Bake for 20 to 30 minutes, until crispy, using a spatula to mix them around on the baking sheet halfway through. Serve warm.

Store cooled leftovers in an airtight container in the refrigerator for 3 to 5 days.

Notes: This recipe is so versatile. If you don't like Old Bay®, you can swap in 1 tablespoon total of mixed spices, like a combo of salt, pepper, and garlic powder—use whatever you have on hand!

You can skip cooking these if you want to dig in right away. Just toss the chickpeas with the oil and Old Bay®, and enjoy. They are delicious served cold!

Sheet Pan Roasted Root Veggies

Serves 8

This is the perfect side dish to accompany your dinner if you are aiming to keep your sugar cravings at bay. Packed with nutritious root veggies, this sheet pan side provides healthy starches without the sugar crash. This recipe is for a big batch—make it on the weekend, and you will have a healthy veggie side to accompany your meals throughout the week.

INGREDIENTS

4 large carrots, cut into 1½-inch pieces

4 medium parsnips, peeled and cut into 1½-inch pieces

3 or 4 golden beets, trimmed, peeled, and cut into wedges

1 pound red potatoes, scrubbed and quartered

1 medium red onion, cut into wedges

½ cup extra-virgin olive oil, plus more as needed

3 tablespoons fresh lemon juice

1 teaspoon fine sea salt

½ teaspoon freshly ground black pepper

½ cup fresh parsley, chopped

3 tablespoons dried rosemary

Preheat the oven to 425°F. Position an oven rack in the center of the oven.

In a large bowl, toss the carrots, parsnips, beets, potatoes, and onion with the olive oil, lemon juice, salt, and pepper. Spread the vegetables in an even layer over two large rimmed baking sheets.

RECIPE CONTINUES

Roast the vegetables for 40 minutes, or until slightly browned around the edges, tossing the vegetables with a rubber spatula half-way through and rotating the pans to avoid burning.

To serve, transfer the roasted vegetables to a large bowl and sprinkle with the parsley and rosemary.

Store leftovers in an airtight container in the refrigerator for up to 4 days.

Note: This is a versatile recipe that works well with many other veggies. Try brussels sprouts, yellow onions, or other types of potatoes.

Sugarless Coffee Creamer

Makes 1¾ cups

I am a coffee person, but I was not a coffee creamer person—until I created this recipe. Coffee creamers can make or break your coffee: they can "make" it by adding delicious flavor to a basic brew, but they can "break" it by being loaded with added sugars. This basic creamer recipe is versatile and can be customized by adding additional extracts or spices to create new flavors. For example, you can use peppermint extract and 1 teaspoon unsweetened cocoa powder for a peppermint mocha creamer.

INGREDIENTS

¾ cup heavy cream

¾ cup unsweetened almond milk

1 teaspoon pure vanilla extract

½ teaspoon pumpkin pie spice, ground cinnamon, peppermint extract, almond extract, or other flavoring of your choice (optional)

In a saucepan, bring ¼ cup water to a rolling boil over medium-high heat. Remove from the heat and pour the water into a heat-safe bowl.

While whisking continuously, slowly add the cream, almond milk, vanilla, and pumpkin pie spice (if using) and whisk until combined. Let cool to room temperature before storing.

Store in an airtight container in the refrigerator for up to 1 week.

Sugarless BBQ Sauce

Makes 1½ cups

Do you often find yourself needing something to dip your food into to jazz it up? I can relate, especially when it comes to boring chicken or salmon. This recipe is for all the big dippers out there. Commercial BBQ sauces have tons of added sugar, but this one has none. With the same core flavors as packaged BBQ sauce, you won't miss the original. Make a batch and store it in the fridge to use as needed for cooking, marinating, and dipping.

INGREDIENTS

¼ small yellow onion, grated

1 large garlic clove, grated

1 (6-ounce) can tomato paste

2 tablespoons apple cider vinegar

2 tablespoons white wine vinegar

2 tablespoons Worcestershire sauce

1 teaspoon chili powder

1 teaspoon fine sea salt

½ teaspoon freshly ground black pepper

½ teaspoon adobo sauce (see Note)

¼ teaspoon ground cinnamon

In a medium saucepan, combine the onion, garlic, tomato paste, apple cider vinegar, white wine vinegar, Worcestershire, chili powder, salt, pepper, adobo sauce, cinnamon, and ⅓ cup water. Bring the mixture to a boil over medium-high heat, then reduce the heat to low. Simmer, uncovered, stirring regularly to prevent sticking, for about 15 minutes, until the mixture begins to thicken. Pour into an airtight container, let cool slightly, and refrigerate for at least 1 hour before using.

Store in the airtight container in the refrigerator for up to 2 weeks.

Notes: Want a thicker sauce? Whisk 1 teaspoon cornstarch into a few table-spoons of water, and then add into the mixture during the last 10 minutes of cooking. This will add a great texture for dipping!

Use the adobo sauce from a can of chipotle peppers in adobo. If you like more heat, you can include a few of the peppers, too.

Sugarless Creamy Caesar Dressing

Makes ½ cup

Many packaged dressings contain added sugar to keep them shelf-stable. By creating your own version, you can avoid the consequences of sugar and its addictive properties. This cashew-based Caesar dressing is creamy and tangy all in one. It's also super simple to make and tastes just like the real thing! You may want to double the recipe—it makes a great dip or topping for other entrées.

INGREDIENTS

½ cup raw cashews

¼ cup fresh lemon juice

2 tablespoons nutritional yeast

1 tablespoon extra-virgin olive oil

1 tablespoon Dijon mustard

2 teaspoons capers

1 garlic clove, minced

Place the cashews in a bowl and cover with 1 cup water. Let soak for 1 to 2 hours, then drain.

Place the soaked cashews in a blender. Blend on high until smooth. Add 2 tablespoons water, the lemon juice, nutritional yeast, olive oil, mustard, capers, and garlic to the blender and blend for about 1 minute, until well combined and smooth.

Store in an airtight container in the refrigerator for up to 1 week.

Notes: If you want a thicker dressing, use less water; for a thinner dressing, add more water 1 tablespoon at a time.

This recipe is vegan, but if you eat meat, try replacing the capers with a few canned sardines. They also contain lots of healthy fatty acids. Just 1½ ounces of sardine has 1 gram of omega-3 fatty acids, one of highest levels of omega-3s found in a low-mercury fish.

Sugarless Ranch Dip

Makes 1 cup

Ranch dressing is a favorite on salads and sandwiches, but it is usually loaded with added sugar. Not this one! This creamy ranch dip is great to serve with your favorite greens or alongside a sandwich (like the Chickpea-Avocado Sandwich on p. 235).

INGREDIENTS

½ cup plain Greek yogurt

½ cup sour cream

1 tablespoon fresh lemon juice

1 tablespoon dried dill

1 tablespoon dried onion flakes

1 teaspoon onion powder

1 teaspoon garlic powder

¼ teaspoon fine sea salt, plus more if needed

¼ teaspoon freshly ground black pepper, plus more if needed

In a small bowl, stir together the yogurt, sour cream, lemon juice, dill, onion flakes, onion powder, garlic powder, salt, and pepper until smooth, about 2 minutes. Taste for seasoning and add more salt and pepper, if needed.

Store in an airtight container in the refrigerator for up to 3 days.

Sugarless Classic Ketchup

Makes 2¼ cups

Ketchup is a staple in most refrigerators, but store-bought varieties can have a ton of added sugar. But not to worry—you can make this simple version at home. The blend of spices complements the tomato—your burgers and fries will thank you!

INGREDIENTS

1 (12-ounce) can tomato paste

½ cup white vinegar

1 teaspoon onion powder

1 teaspoon garlic powder

¾ teaspoon fine sea salt

½ teaspoon paprika

½ teaspoon Worcestershire sauce

¼ teaspoon freshly ground black pepper

⅛ teaspoon ground cloves

⅛ teaspoon ground mustard

In a medium saucepan, combine 1 cup water, the tomato paste, vinegar, onion powder, garlic powder, salt, paprika, Worcestershire, pepper, cloves, and mustard. Bring to a simmer over medium heat, whisking occasionally, about 2 minutes. Cover and reduce the heat to low. Cook for about 15 minutes, until thickened. Remove from the heat and let cool before serving or storing.

Store in an airtight container in the refrigerator for up to 2 weeks.

Strawberry Shortcake Parfait

Serves 3

These individual no-sugar-added strawberry shortcake parfait cups are filling and full of fiber and protein from the oats and yogurt. The mashed banana adds the perfect amount of sweetness, making it a great no-added-sugar recipe. These make a healthy dessert anytime, or prepare them as a weekend breakfast treat. You can add another layer of yogurt and strawberry on top if you are looking for a little more to eat!

INGREDIENTS

For the shortcakes

1½ cups oat flour (see Notes)

¼ teaspoon baking soda

¼ teaspoon ground cinnamon

Pinch of fine sea salt

¼ cup mashed banana

1 large egg

¼ cup milk of choice

2 tablespoons unsalted butter or butter substitute, melted

1 teaspoon pure vanilla extract

For the parfaits

1 cup yogurt of choice (see Notes)

1 cup quartered strawberries

RECIPE CONTINUES

MAKE THE SHORTCAKES: Preheat the oven to 350°F. Line six wells of a muffin tin with paper liners.

In a medium bowl, whisk together the oat flour, baking soda, cinnamon, and salt. In another bowl, stir together the banana, egg, milk, melted butter, and vanilla. Fold the wet mixture into the dry mixture just enough to combine.

Fill each lined well of the muffin tin with ¼ cup of the batter. Bake for 20 to 25 minutes, until a toothpick inserted into the center of a shortcake comes out clean. Remove from the pan and refrigerate the shortcakes for 25 minutes, or until cooled.

ASSEMBLE THE PARFAITS: Crumble one shortcake into the bottom of a 1-pint mason jar, then add ⅓ cup of the yogurt, ⅓ cup of the strawberries, and one more crumbled shortcake on top. Repeat to assemble two more parfaits.

You may store the shortcakes in an airtight container in the refrigerator for 2 to 3 days. Store the strawberries and yogurt separately and build the parfait just before serving to prevent sogginess.

Notes: To make oat flour at home, blend oats in a high-speed blender for 1 minute, or until they have been ground super fine.

Try replacing the mashed banana with no-sugar-added applesauce or pure pumpkin puree, which could be a great swap during the holiday seasons!

For the yogurt, you can use plain or vanilla Greek yogurt, or try a plant-based alternative like coconut yogurt, almond yogurt, or soy yogurt. Just be sure to check the labels to ensure that there isn't any added sugar.

Frozen Yogurt Bark with Nuts and Berries

Serves 4

This healthy frozen yogurt bark is simple to make and will become the guilt-free answer to your sweet cravings! You can make up a few batches of these to keep on hand in your freezer as a healthy—and sugarless—sweet treat. The best thing about this recipe is that the toppings are completely customizable based on your preferences. You can switch out the nuts for seeds and the cacao nibs for coconut flakes, if you like.

INGREDIENTS

    1 cup unsweetened vanilla yogurt (see Notes)

    ¼ cup chopped nuts of your choice (see Notes)

    ¼ cup whole raspberries, chopped strawberries, halved
        blackberries, or whole blueberries

    1 tablespoon cacao nibs

Line a 9-inch square baking pan with parchment paper. Spoon the yogurt into the lined pan and spread it out into an even layer, about ¼ inch thick (it will not cover the whole surface of the pan). Sprinkle the nuts evenly over the yogurt, followed by the berries and cacao nibs. Freeze for 1 hour before serving. To serve, break up the bark into smaller pieces.

    Store, covered, in the freezer for 1 to 2 weeks.

Notes: Any type of yogurt will work. I recommend coconut yogurt, Greek yogurt, oat milk yogurt, or soy yogurt. For the nuts, I recommend almonds, pistachios, or cashews.

Salted Caramel-ish Rice Puff Bars

Makes 9 bars

Craving a frozen dessert? These bars satisfy that sweet and salty aspect while being perfectly cold, crunchy, and—best yet—sugarless! Although they don't technically contain caramel, the ingredients blend together to look and taste just like it. When stored in the freezer, they keep for weeks, and are great to have on hand for when you are craving something sweet.

INGREDIENTS

3 tablespoons coconut oil, melted

⅓ cup unsweetened creamy almond, cashew, or peanut butter

¼ cup unsweetened applesauce (see Notes)

¼ teaspoon ground cinnamon

1 teaspoon pure vanilla extract

2 cups plain puffed rice or crushed rice cakes

Pinch of fine sea salt

Line a 9-inch square baking pan with parchment paper.

In a medium saucepan, combine the melted coconut oil, nut butter, applesauce, cinnamon, and vanilla. Cook over medium heat, stirring occasionally, until the mixture is thick and warmed through, about 3 minutes. Remove from the heat and fold in the puffed rice until thoroughly coated.

Pour the mixture into the prepared pan and use a rubber spatula to spread it into an even layer. Top with the salt and freeze for 30 minutes. Remove from the freezer and cut into 9 equal-size bars.

Store, covered, in the freezer for up to 3 weeks. Keep them frozen until ready to serve, then allow them to thaw for 5 minutes before eating.

Notes: Make sure the applesauce you use is not too watery, or the bars may fall apart. If your applesauce appears watery, cook the mixture longer to evaporate some of the moisture before stirring in the puffed rice. An alternative to applesauce is mashed banana.

This recipe is very versatile. You can add in other ingredients to boost the nutritional value, including chia seeds, hemp seeds, oats, coconut shavings, and dried fruit. If desired, melt some of your favorite 100 percent cacao dark chocolate (without any added sugar, stevia, or artificial sugars) and drizzle it over the top.

Blueberry Oatmeal Muffins

Makes 8 muffins

I love muffins, but the ones you find at the store are basically cake disguised as something supposedly healthy. It is almost impossible to find store-bought muffins without added sugar, so I make my own. You can use any type of fruit, but frozen or fresh blueberries are my go-to. Frozen wild blueberries are a great option, as they have twice the antioxidants as regular blueberries and are also known to help reduce cravings for sugar—an added bonus!

INGREDIENTS:

1¼ cups rolled oats

½ cup unsweetened coconut flakes

½ teaspoon baking soda

¼ teaspoon fine sea salt

½ cup mashed banana or unsweetened applesauce

¼ cup milk of choice

2 large eggs

1 teaspoon pure vanilla extract

1 cup fresh or frozen blueberries (see Notes)

Preheat the oven to 350°F. Line eight wells of a muffin tin with paper liners.

In a blender, combine the oats and coconut and blend to a fine powder, about 30 seconds (see Notes). Transfer the mixture to a medium bowl and stir in the baking soda and salt. In another bowl, mix the banana, milk, eggs, and vanilla. Add the dry ingredients to the wet ingredients and mix just until combined, then gently fold in the blueberries.

Divide the batter among the lined wells of the muffin tin, using about ⅓ cup for each. Bake for about 20 minutes, until golden, soft, and fluffy. Let cool before serving or storing.

Store in an airtight container in the refrigerator for 4 to 5 days (see Notes).

Notes: If you use frozen blueberries, the blueberry color will transfer to the batter, but fresh blueberries won't have any color transfer. Either way, they taste amazing.

Do not overblend the oats and coconut, or the coconut will start to secrete its oils. This will make the mixture dense and too hard to mix into the batter.

If the muffins have been in the fridge, I recommend popping them into the microwave for 10 to 15 seconds or into a hot oven for 2 to 3 minutes before eating so they are warm!

Whole-Fruit Frozen Rocket Pops

Makes 8 pops

My favorite summertime childhood treat was when my mom would let my brother and me get something from the ice-cream truck—and I would always choose a rocket pop! Those pops I ate back in the '80s were loaded with sugar, but fear not—I have re-created them! Summertime calls for ice pops, but not the sugar-filled ones from the store or the ice-cream truck. These homemade whole-fruit rocket pops are the perfect sunny-day treat, and this recipe makes a full week's worth of frozen sweet treats for the whole family. And in addition to being free of added sugar, these rocket pops contain loads of nutrients and fiber that typical ice pops lack.

INGREDIENTS

1 cup stemmed strawberries

1 teaspoon lime zest

3 tablespoons fresh lime juice (from 2 limes)

⅓ cup canned unsweetened coconut milk, full-fat or lower-fat (see Note)

⅓ cup sliced banana

1½ teaspoons grated fresh ginger

1 cup blueberries

2 teaspoons finely chopped fresh mint

In a blender, combine the strawberries, lime zest, and 2 tablespoons of the lime juice and blend until smooth. Pour the mixture evenly into eight 2½-ounce rocket pop molds (about 4 teaspoons for each). Cover the molds with plastic wrap and freeze until just set, 45 minutes to 1 hour.

Meanwhile, rinse your blender clean. Combine the coconut milk, banana, and ginger in the clean blender and blend until smooth. Remove the molds from the freezer and pour the coconut milk mixture evenly over the strawberry mixture in each mold (use about 4 teaspoons for each) to form a second layer. Cover with the plastic wrap and freeze again until just set, 45 minutes to 1 hour.

Meanwhile, rinse your blender clean one last time. Combine the blueberries, mint, and remaining 1 tablespoon lime juice in the clean blender and blend until smooth. Remove the molds from the freezer and pour the blueberry mixture evenly over the coconut mixture in each mold (use about 4 teaspoons for each) to form a third layer. Insert ice pop sticks into each pop and freeze completely, about 4 hours.

To serve, run the molds under warm water for a few seconds, then gently pull the pops out of their molds.

Store the ice pops in their molds in the freezer for up to 6 months.

Note: If you're not a huge fan of coconut milk, opt for unsweetened Greek yogurt. Use about 1 cup yogurt mixed with 2 to 3 tablespoons water to give your pop the same creamy texture it would have if you had used coconut milk.

Unbelievable Ice Cream Sundae

Serves 2

You have heard of the Impossible Burger®, right? Well, meet the Unbelievable Ice Cream Sundae. All the joys of your favorite ice cream sundae, without the sugar. The ice cream itself is made from bananas, which are packed with fiber and nutrients to prevent our bodies from experiencing spikes in blood sugar. This means that instead of getting an ice cream sugar high, you'll feel energized and ready to take on the day.

INGREDIENTS

2 large bananas, peeled, sliced, and frozen

½ teaspoon pure vanilla extract

1 (14.5-ounce) can unsweetened full-fat coconut milk, chilled overnight

2 tablespoons unsweetened raw cacao powder

1½ tablespoons coconut oil, melted

2 tablespoons unsweetened creamy peanut butter

Optional toppings

Crushed banana chips

Crushed walnuts

Cacao nibs

Fresh berries (see Note)

Put the frozen banana in a food processor and process on high until smooth and creamy, scraping down the sides and adding 1 tablespoon water as needed. Add the vanilla and process until combined.

Transfer the banana ice cream to a freezer-safe container and freeze for at least 1 hour before serving.

While the ice cream is setting in the freezer, open the chilled can of coconut milk and scoop the solid white portion into a large bowl, leaving the watery liquid in the can to save for another use, if you like. Using a handheld mixer, beat the coconut cream until fluffy, 30 to 60 seconds. Refrigerate the whipped cream until you're ready to assemble the sundaes.

In a small bowl, whisk together the cacao powder and melted coconut oil until smooth. Set the chocolate sauce aside at room temperature until ready to serve (do not chill or the coconut oil will harden).

In a small bowl, stir together the peanut butter and 2 to 3 table-spoons water, adding the water 1 tablespoon at a time until you get a smooth consistency. Set the peanut butter sauce aside at room temperature until ready to serve.

To serve, divide the banana ice cream between two sundae dishes. Top each with a large dollop of the whipped cream, a drizzle of the chocolate sauce, and another of the peanut butter sauce, then finish with your desired toppings.

Store leftover ice cream in a freezer-safe container in the freezer for up to 1 month. The whipped cream, chocolate sauce, and peanut butter sauce don't store well, so use them right away and remake them as needed for serving.

Note: For a great crunchy topping, try dehydrated fruit, like bananas, straw-berries, blueberries, or apples. Dehydrated versions of all these fruits and more are affordable alternatives to fresh fruit and last a longer time in your pantry. They also make a great snack by themselves.

Easy Flaxseed Crackers with Olive Hummus

Makes about 8 servings

If you are looking for a sugarless snack that will satisfy your craving for something crunchy, these flax crackers with olive-topped hummus are a must-try. Flaxseeds are high in healthy fats, as well as fiber, which will be helpful in reducing your cravings. If you want something on the sweeter side, try pairing these crackers with natural peanut butter instead of the olive hummus.

INGREDIENTS

For the crackers

1 cup flaxseed meal (see Note)

1 tablespoon extra-virgin olive oil

1 teaspoon fine sea salt

1 teaspoon white sesame seeds

¼ teaspoon freshly ground black pepper

¼ teaspoon garlic powder

For the hummus

3½ cups canned chickpeas (two 15-ounce cans), drained and rinsed

½ cup tahini

¼ cup extra-virgin olive oil, plus more for serving

¼ cup fresh lemon juice

3 garlic cloves, peeled

1 teaspoon fine sea salt

⅓ cup chopped pitted kalamata olives

MAKE THE CRACKERS: Preheat the oven to 350°F.

In a large bowl, stir together the flaxseed meal, olive oil, salt, sesame seeds, pepper, garlic powder, and ¼ cup water until well combined. The texture should be slightly crumbly, but if it is too crumbly, you can add a little extra water or olive oil 1 tablespoon at a time.

Place the dough between two pieces of parchment paper and roll it out into a thin rectangle, about 12 by 9 inches and ⅛ inch thick. If you don't have an even-looking rectangle, just use a pizza cutter or knife to square off the sides, place the scraps in the middle of the rectangle, and roll it out some more.

Peel off the top piece of parchment paper. Slide the bottom piece of parchment with the rolled-out dough onto a large baking sheet. Using a knife or pizza cutter, score a grid pattern in the dough to form 1½-inch square crackers. (Don't cut all the way through—you will break the crackers apart along the scored lines after baking.)

Bake until the crackers are lightly browned, 18 to 20 minutes, keeping an eye on them so they don't start to burn. Let cool completely, then break apart along the scored lines to form individual crackers.

WHILE THE CRACKERS ARE COOLING, MAKE THE HUMMUS: In a food processor, combine the chickpeas, tahini, olive oil, lemon juice, garlic, salt, and ¼ cup water. Process until smooth, 3 to 4 minutes, stopping to scrape the sides as needed. If the hummus is too thick, add water 1 tablespoon at a time until it reaches the desired consistency.

For the olives, you have two options: you can incorporate the olives into the hummus by adding them to the mixture while it is still in the food processor and pulsing 6 or 7 times, then transfer to a serving bowl;

RECIPE CONTINUES

or you can transfer the hummus to a serving bowl and add the olives on top. Either way, refrigerate the hummus for at least 1 hour before serving.

Garnish the hummus with a splash of olive oil and more chopped olives, if desired. Serve alongside the crackers.

Store the hummus in an airtight container in the refrigerator for up to 3 days. Store the crackers in an airtight container at room temperature for 3 to 4 days.

Note: The easiest option is to buy flax meal preground, but you can grind your own using a blender, food processor, or even a coffee grinder. If you choose to grind your own, golden flaxseeds work best.

DIFFERENT NAMES FOR ADDED SUGAR

1. Agave nectar
2. Agave syrup
3. Anhydrous dextrose
4. Apple juice concentrate
5. Barley malt
6. Barley malt extract
7. Barley malt syrup
8. Beet juice concentrate
9. Beet sugar
10. Beet syrup
11. Blackberry juice concentrate
12. Blackcurrant juice concentrate
13. Blackstrap molasses
14. Blood orange juice concentrate
15. Blueberry juice concentrate
16. Boysenberry juice concentrate
17. Brown cane sugar
18. Brown rice syrup
19. Brown rice syrup solids
20. Brown sugar
21. Brown sugar syrup
22. Cane crystals
23. Cane juice
24. Cane juice crystals
25. Cane molasses
26. Cane refinery syrup
27. Cane sugar
28. Cane syrup
29. Caramelized pear juice concentrate
30. Caramelized sugar
31. Caramelized sugar syrup
32. Carrot juice concentrate
33. Cherry juice concentrate
34. Clarified guava juice concentrate
35. Clarified lime juice concentrate
36. Clover honey
37. Coconut blossom sugar
38. Coconut nectar
39. Coconut palm nectar
40. Coconut palm sugar
41. Coconut sugar
42. Coconut sugar crystals
43. Concentrated melon juice
44. Corn barley malt syrup
45. Corn dextrin
46. Corn maltodextrin
47. Corn sweetener
48. Corn syrup
49. Corn syrup butter
50. Corn syrup solids
51. Cranberry juice concentrate
52. Crystalline fructose
53. Dark brown cane sugar
54. Dark brown sugar
55. Date crystals
56. Date juice concentrate

57. Date syrup
58. Decorative sugars
59. Dehydrated cane juice
60. Dehydrated cane sugar
61. Demerara sugar
62. Dextrin
63. Dextrose
64. Dextrose anhydrous glucose
65. Dextrose sugar
66. Diastatic malt
67. Diastatic malt powder
68. Dried brown rice syrup
69. Dried cane sugar
70. Dried cane syrup
71. Dried cherry juice concentrate
72. Dried corn syrup
73. Dried cranberry juice concentrate
74. Dried glucose syrup
75. Elderberry juice concentrate
76. Ethyl maltol
77. Evaporated cane crystals
78. Evaporated cane juice
79. Evaporated cane juice invert syrup
80. Evaporated cane sugar
81. Evaporated cane syrup
82. Evaporated coconut palm nectar
83. Fair trade unrefined cane sugar
84. Fondant sugar
85. Fructan
86. Fructooligosaccharides
87. Fructose
88. Fructose syrup
89. Fruit juice concentrate
90. Galactooligosaccharides
91. Glucose
92. Glucose fructose syrup
93. Glucose solids
94. Glucose syrup
95. Glucose syrup solids
96. Goji berry juice concentrate
97. Golden brown sugar
98. Golden sugar
99. Golden syrup
100. Granulated sugar
101. Grape juice concentrate
102. Grape sugar
103. Grapefruit juice concentrate
104. High fructose corn syrup
105. High maltose corn syrup solids
106. Honey
107. Honey powder
108. Honeydew juice concentrate
109. Icing sugar
110. Invert cane sugar
111. Invert cane syrup
112. Invert sugar
113. Invert sugar cane syrup
114. Invert sugar syrup
115. Invert syrup
116. Isomalto-oligosaccharide
117. Key lime juice concentrate
118. Kiwi juice concentrate
119. Lactose
120. Lemon juice concentrate
121. Light brown cane sugar

122. Light brown sugar
123. Liquid sugar
124. Loganberry juice concentrate
125. Malt extract
126. Malt syrup
127. Maltodextrin
128. Maltol
129. Maltose
130. Mango juice concentrate
131. Maple sugar
132. Maple syrup
133. Melon juice concentrate
134. Milled cane sugar
135. Molasses
136. Molasses granules
137. Molasses powder
138. Monk fruit juice concentrate
139. Monk juice concentrate
140. Muscovado
141. Non-GMO honey
142. Oat syrup solids
143. Orange juice concentrate
144. Organic agave nectar
145. Organic agave syrup
146. Organic apple juice concentrate
147. Organic barley malt syrup
148. Organic blueberry juice concentrate
149. Organic brown rice syrup
150. Organic brown sugar
151. Organic cane crystals
152. Organic cane sugar
153. Organic cane syrup
154. Organic cherry juice concentrate
155. Organic coconut blossom nectar
156. Organic coconut nectar
157. Organic coconut palm nectar
158. Organic coconut palm sugar
159. Organic coconut sugar
160. Organic coconut syrup
161. Organic corn syrup solids
162. Organic date nectar
163. Organic date sugar
164. Organic date syrup
165. Organic dextrose
166. Organic dried cane sugar
167. Organic dried cane syrup
168. Organic dried cherry juice concentrate
169. Organic dried cranberry juice concentrate
170. Organic evaporated cane juice
171. Organic evaporated cane juice syrup
172. Organic evaporated coconut palm nectar
173. Organic fair trade unrefined cane sugar
174. Organic fruit juice concentrate
175. Organic glucose syrup
176. Organic grape juice concentrate
177. Organic honey
178. Organic invert cane sugar
179. Organic invert cane syrup
180. Organic invert sugar
181. Organic invert sugar cane syrup

182. Organic invert sugar syrup

183. Organic invert syrup

184. Organic lactose

185. Organic lemon juice concentrate

186. Organic light brown sugar

187. Organic maltodextrin

188. Organic maple syrup

189. Organic milled cane sugar

190. Organic molasses

191. Organic molasses granules

192. Organic non-GMO honey

193. Organic panela sugar

194. Organic pineapple juice concentrate

195. Organic powdered sugar

196. Organic raisin juice concentrate

197. Organic raw dark agave syrup

198. Organic raw honey

199. Organic rice maltodextrin

200. Organic rice syrup

201. Organic rice syrup solids

202. Organic strawberry juice concentrate

203. Organic sugar

204. Organic sugar cane syrup

205. Organic yapioca maltodextrin

206. Organic tapioca syrup

207. Organic tapioca syrup solids

208. Organic white grape juice concentrate

209. Palm sugar

210. Passion fruit juice concentrate

211. Peach juice concentrate

212. Pear juice concentrate

213. Pear syrup

214. Pineapple juice concentrate

215. Pineapple syrup

216. Plum juice concentrate

217. Pomegranate juice concentrate

218. Powdered sugar

219. Pure cane golden brown sugar

220. Pure cane sugar

221. Pure local sorghum molasses

222. Pure maple syrup

223. Raisin juice concentrate

224. Raisin nectar

225. Raspberry juice concentrate

226. Raw cane sugar

227. Raw honey

228. Raw sugar

229. Refiner's syrup

230. Refinery syrup

231. Rice maltodextrin

232. Rice syrup

233. Rice syrup solids

234. Saccharose

235. Sorghum syrup

236. Strawberry juice concentrate

237. Sucrose

238. Sugar

239. Sugar beet syrup

240. Sugar cane syrup

241. Sugarcane molasses

242. Syrup

243. Tapioca dextrin

244. Tapioca maltodextrin

245. Tapioca syrup
246. Tapioca syrup solids
247. Tart cherry juice concentrate
248. Treacle
249. Trehalose
250. Turbinado sugar
251. Unsulfured molasses
252. Watermelon juice concentrate

253. Wheat dextrin
254. Wheat glucose syrup
255. White grain sorghum extract
256. White granulated sugar
257. White grape juice concentrate
258. White sugar
259. Wildflower honey

Worksheets for the 7-Step Plan to Uncover Hidden Sugars, Curb Your Cravings, and Conquer Your Addiction

These worksheets will help you navigate the steps for breaking your addiction to sugar outlined in chapter 4.

Fridge/Pantry

Item	Brand

Grams of Added Sugar	Alternative Sweeteners (Yes/No)	Type of Alternative Sweetener

3-Day Food Diary

Day 1

Food Item	Grams of Added Sugar	Time of Day

Day 2

Food Item	Grams of Added Sugar	Time of Day

Day 3

Food Item	Grams of Added Sugar	Time of Day

Dining Out

Name of Restaurant	Food(s) Ordered	Time of Day

ARE YOU ADDICTED TO SUGAR?

For the following questions, please answer yes or no.

In the past 12 months:

1. When offered something sweet, I usually eat it.

2. When eating something with sugar in it I normally have more than one serving.

3. If I am emotional, I eat something with sugar in it to feel better.

4. I eat foods with sugar to the point where it makes me physically ill.

5. I continue to eat foods with sugar even though I know it has caused emotional problems for me.

6. I have strong desires for foods with sugars to the point where I am unable to concentrate on anything else.

7. I have avoided situations where I knew there would be foods with sugars because I knew I would overindulge on them.

8. I have tried to reduce or stop how much sugar I eat but I have been unable to do so.

9. I was distracted by thinking about sugar to the point where I could have been seriously injured or hurt (e.g., while crossing a street, driving a car, cooking).

10. How much and how often I eat sugar has made me upset.

11. I have had significant problems with my life (e.g., family, friends, work, daily routine, physical/mental health) because of sugar.

12. My friends or family have expressed concern over how much I eat sugar.

13. I often feel extremely tired after eating sugar.

Scoring:

If you answered YES to

0–1 question = no addiction
2–3 questions = mild addiction
4–5 questions = moderate addiction
6 or more questions = severe addiction

Adapted from Yale Food Addiction Scale.
https://sites.lsa.umich.edu/fastlab/yale-food-addiction-scale/

REFERENCES

INTRODUCTION

Keys, A., Taylor, H. L., Blackburn, H., Brozek, J., Anderson, J. T., and Simonson, E. (1963). Coronary Heart Disease among Minnesota Business and Professional Men Followed Fifteen Years. *Circulation*, 28(3), 381–395. https://doi.org/10.1161/01.cir.28.3.381

CHAPTER 1

AlEssa, H. B., Bhupathiraju, S. N., Malik, V. S., Wedick, N. M., Campos, H., Rosner, B., Willett, W. C., and Hu, F. B. (2015). Carbohydrate Quality and Quantity and Risk of Type 2 Diabetes in US Women. *The American Journal of Clinical Nutrition*, 102(6), 1543–1553. https://doi.org/10.3945/ajcn.115.116558

Any Anxiety Disorder. (n.d.) *National Institute of Mental Health (NIMH)*. Accessed July 31, 2022. https://www.nimh.nih.gov/health/statistics/any-anxiety-disorder#part_2576

Appleton, J. (2018). The Gut-Brain Axis: Influence of Microbiota on Mood and Mental Health. *Integrative Medicine* (Encinitas, Calif.), 17(4), 28–32.

Atkinson, F. S., Foster-Powell, K., and Brand-Miller, J. C. (2008). International Tables of Glycemic Index and Glycemic Load Values: 2008. *Diabetes Care*, 31(12), 2281–2283. https://doi.org/10.2337/dc08-1239

Bahniwal, M., Little, J. P., and Klegeris, A. (2017). High Glucose Enhances Neurotoxicity and Inflammatory Cytokine Secretion by Stimulated Human Astrocytes. *Current Alzheimer Research*, 14(7), 731–741. https://doi.org/10.2174/1567205014666170117104053

Basu, A. K. (2018). DNA Damage, Mutagenesis and Cancer. *International Journal of Molecular Sciences*, 19(4), 970. https://doi.org/10.3390/ijms19040970

Basu, R. (2019, April 19). Type 2 Diabetes. *NIDDK. National Institute of Diabetes and Digestive and Kidney Diseases*. Accessed July 31, 2022. https://www.niddk.nih.gov/health-information/diabetes/overview/what-is-diabetes/type-2-diabetes

Bays, H. E., Kulkarni, A., German, C., Satish, P., Iluyomade, A., Dudum, R., Thakkar, A., Rifai, M. A., Mehta, A., Thobani, A., Al-Saiegh, Y., Nelson, A. J., Sheth, S., and Toth, P. P. (2022). Ten Things to Know about Ten Cardiovascular Disease Risk Factors (2022). *American Journal of Preventive Cardiology*, 10, 100342. https://doi.org/10.1016/j.ajpc.2022.100342

Berger, P. K., Plows, J. F., Jones, R. B., Alderete, T. L., Rios, C., Pickering, T. A., Fields, D. A., Bode, L., Peterson, B. S., and Goran, M. I. (2020). Associations of Maternal Fructose and Sugar-Sweetened Beverage and Juice Intake during Lactation with Infant Neurodevelopmental Outcomes at 24 Months. *The American Journal of Clinical Nutrition*, 112(6), 1516–1522. https://doi.org/10.1093/ajcn/nqaa255

Berlanga-Acosta, J., Guillén-Nieto, G., Rodríguez-Rodríguez, N., Bringas-Vega, M. L., García-Del-Barco-Herrera, D., Berlanga-Saez, J. O., García-Ojalvo, A., Valdés-Sosa, M. J., and Valdés-Sosa, P. A. (2020). Insulin Resistance at the Crossroad of Alzheimer Disease Pathology: A Review. *Frontiers in Endocrinology*, 11, 560375. https://doi.org/10.3389/fendo.2020.560375

References

Biederman, J., Petty, C. R., Evans, M., Small, J., and Faraone, S. V. (2010). How Persistent Is ADHD? A Controlled 10-Year Follow-Up Study of Boys with ADHD. *Psychiatry Research*, 177(3), 299–304. https://doi.org/10.1016/j.psychres.2009.12.010

Brand-Miller, J., Hayne, S., Petocz, P., and Colagiuri, S. (2003). Low-Glycemic Index Diets in the Management of Diabetes: A Meta-Analysis of Randomized Controlled Trials. *Diabetes Care*, 26(8), 2261–2267. https://doi.org/10.2337/diacare.26.8.2261

Breymeyer, K. L., Lampe, J. W., McGregor, B. A., and Neuhouser, M. L. (2016). Subjective Mood and Energy Levels of Healthy Weight and Overweight/Obese Healthy Adults on High- and Low-Glycemic Load Experimental Diets. *Appetite*, 107, 253–259. https://doi.org/10.1016/j.appet.2016.08.008

CDC. (2019, October 3). *On Your Way to Preventing Type 2 Diabetes*. Centers for Disease Control and Prevention. https://www.cdc.gov/diabetes/prevent-type-2/guide-prevent-type2-diabetes.html

———. (2021, September 27). *Heart Disease Facts*. Centers for Disease Control and Prevention. https://www.cdc.gov/heartdisease/facts.htm

———. (2016, January 1). *Cancers Associated with Overweight and Obesity Make up 40 percent of Cancers Diagnosed in the United States*. Centers for Disease Control and Prevention. https://www.cdc.gov/media/releases/2017/p1003-vs-cancer-obesity.html

Cetinkalp, S., Simsir, I. Y., and Ertek, S. (2014). Insulin Resistance in Brain and Possible Therapeutic Approaches. *Current Vascular Pharmacology*, 12(4), 553–564. https://doi.org/10.2174/1570161112999914020613042

Chong, C. P., Shahar, S., Haron, H., and Din, N. C. (2019). Habitual Sugar Intake and Cognitive Impairment among Multi-Ethnic Malaysian Older Adults. *Clinical Interventions in Aging*, 14, 1331–1342. https://doi.org/10.2147/CIA.S211534

Cohen, J., Rifas-Shiman, S. L., Young, J., and Oken, E. (2018). Associations of Prenatal and Child Sugar Intake with Child Cognition. *American Journal of Preventive Medicine*, 54(6), 727–735. https://doi.org/10.1016/j.amepre.2018.02.020

Coletro, H. N., Mendonça, R. D., Meireles, A. L., Machado-Coelho, G., and Menezes, M. C. (2022). Ultra-Processed and Fresh Food Consumption and Symptoms of Anxiety and Depression during the COVID-19 Pandemic: COVID Inconfidentes. *Clinical Nutrition ESPEN*, 47, 206–214. https://doi.org/10.1016/j.clnesp.2021.12.013

Debras, C., Chazelas, E., Srour, B., Kesse-Guyot, E., Julia, C., Zelek, L., Agaësse, C., Druesne-Pecollo, N., Galan, P., Hercberg, S., Latino-Martel, P., Deschasaux, M., and Touvier, M. (2020). Total and Added Sugar Intakes, Sugar Types, and Cancer Risk: Results from the Prospective NutriNet-Santé Cohort. *The American Journal of Clinical Nutrition*, 112(5), 1267–1279. https://doi.org/10.1093/ajcn/nqaa246

Del-Ponte, B., Anselmi, L., Assunção, M., Tovo-Rodrigues, L., Munhoz, T. N., Matijasevich, A., Rohde, L. A., and Santos, I. S. (2019). Sugar Consumption and Attention-Deficit/Hyperactivity Disorder (ADHD): A Birth Cohort Study. *Journal of Affective Disorders*, 243, 290–296. https://doi.org/10.1016/j.jad.2018.09.051

Duan, M.-J., Vinke, P. C., Navis, G., Corpeleijn, E., and Dekker, L. H. (2022). Ultra-Processed Food and Incident Type 2 Diabetes: Studying the Underlying Consumption Patterns to Unravel the Health Effects of This Heterogeneous Food Category in the Prospective Lifelines Cohort. *BMC Medicine*, 20(1). https://doi.org/10.1186/s12916-021-02200-4

References

Dunn, G. A., Nigg, J. T., and Sullivan, E. L. (2019). Neuroinflammation as a Risk Factor for Attention Deficit Hyperactivity Disorder. *Pharmacology, Biochemistry, and Behavior*, 182, 22–34. https://doi.org/10.1016/j.pbb.2019.05.005

Farsad-Naeimi, A., Asjodi, F., Omidian, M., Askari, M., Nouri, M., Pizarro, A. B., and Daneshzad, E. (2020). Sugar Consumption, Sugar Sweetened Beverages and Attention Deficit Hyperactivity Disorder: A Systematic Review and Meta-Analysis. *Complementary Therapies in Medicine*, 53, 102512. https://doi.org/10.1016/j.ctim.2020.102512

Faruque, S., Tong, J., Lacmanovic, V., Agbonghae, C., Minaya, D. M., and Czaja, K. (2019). The Dose Makes the Poison: Sugar and Obesity in the United States—a Review. *Polish Journal of Food and Nutrition Sciences*, 69(3), 219–233. https://doi.org/10.31883/pjfns/110735

Finch, L. E., and Tomiyama, A. J. (2015b). Comfort Eating, Psychological Stress, and Depressive Symptoms in Young Adult Women. *Appetite*, 95, 239–244. https://doi.org/10.1016/j.appet.2015.07.017

Gorelick, P. B. (2010). Role of Inflammation in Cognitive Impairment: Results of Observational Epidemiological Studies and Clinical Trials. *Annals of the New York Academy of Sciences*, 1207, 155–162. https://doi.org/10.1111/j.1749-6632.2010.05726.x

Hamel, V., Nardocci, M., Flexner, N., Bernstein, J., L'Abbé, M. R., and Moubarac, J.-C. (2022). Consumption of Ultra-Processed Foods Is Associated with Free Sugars Intake in the Canadian Population. *Nutrients*, 14(3), 708. https://doi.org/10.3390/nu14030708

Harvard Public Health. (2013). Added Sugar in the Diet. *The Nutrition Source*. Accessed March 8, 2022. https://www.hsph.harvard.edu/nutritionsource/carbohydrates/added-sugar-in-the-diet/#:~:text=The%20average%20American%20consumes%2022

Howard, A. L., Robinson, M., Smith, G. J., Ambrosini, G. L., Piek, J. P., and Oddy, W. H. (2011). ADHD Is Associated with a "Western" Dietary Pattern in Adolescents. *Journal of Attention Disorders*, 15(5), 403–411. https://doi.org/10.1177/1087054710365990

Hsieh, C. F., Liu, C. K., Lee, C. T., Yu, L. E., and Wang, J. Y. (2019). Acute Glucose Fluctuation Impacts Microglial Activity, Leading to Inflammatory Activation or Self-Degradation. *Scientific Reports*, 9(1), 840. https://doi.org/10.1038/s41598-018-37215-0

Huang, Y., Chen, Z., Chen, B., Li, J., Yuan, X., Li, J., Wang, W., Dai, T., Chen, H., Wang, Y., Wang, R., Wang, P., Guo, J., Dong, Q., Liu, C., Wei, Q., Cao, D., and Liu, L. (2023). Dietary Sugar Consumption and Health: Umbrella Review. *BMJ*, 5, 381:e071609. doi: 10.1136/bmj-2022-071609. PMID: 37019448

Jacka, F. N., Cherbuin, N., Anstey, K. J., Sachdev, P., and Butterworth, P. (2015). Western Diet Is Associated with a Smaller Hippocampus: A Longitudinal Investigation. *BMC Medicine*, 13, 215. https://doi.org/10.1186/s12916-015-0461-x

Johnson, R. J., Sánchez-Lozada, L. G., Andrews, P., and Lanaspa, M. A. (2017). Perspective: A Historical and Scientific Perspective of Sugar and Its Relation with Obesity and Diabetes. *Advances in Nutrition* (Bethesda, Md.), 8(3), 412–422. https://doi.org/10.3945/an.116.014654

Kaaks, R., and Lukanova, A. (2001). Energy Balance and Cancer: The Role of Insulin and Insulin-Like Growth Factor-I. *The Proceedings of the Nutrition Society*, 60(1), 91–106. https://doi.org/10.1079/pns200070

Kendzor, D. E., Chen, M., Reininger, B. M., Businelle, M. S., Stewart, D. W., Fisher-Hoch, S. P., Rentfro, A. R., Wetter, D. W., and McCormick, J. B. (2014). The Association of Depression and Anxiety with Glycemic Control among Mexican Americans with Diabetes Living near the U.S.–Mexico Border. *BMC Public Health*, 14, 176. https://doi.org/10.1186/1471-2458-14-176

References

Kose, J., Cheung, A., Fezeu, L. K., Péneau, S., Debras, C., Touvier, M., Hercberg, S., Galan, P., and Andreeva, V. A. (2021). A Comparison of Sugar Intake between Individuals with High and Low Trait Anxiety: Results from the NutriNet-Santé Study. *Nutrients*, 13(5), 1526. https://doi .org/10.3390/nu13051526

Kouvari, M., D'Cunha, N. M., Travica, N., Sergi, D., Zec, M., Marx, W., and Naumovski, N. (2022). Metabolic Syndrome, Cognitive Impairment and the Role of Diet: A Narrative Review. *Nutrients*, 14(2), 333. https://doi.org/10.3390/nu14020333

Kvalvik, L. G., Klungsøyr, K., Igland, J., Caspersen, I. H., Brantsæter, A. L., Solberg, B. S., Hartman, C., Schweren, L., Larsson, H., Li, L., Forthun, I., Johansson, S., Arias Vasquez, A., and Haavik, J. (2022). Association of Sweetened Carbonated Beverage Consumption during Pregnancy and ADHD Symptoms in the Offspring: A Study from the Norwegian Mother, Father and Child Cohort Study (MoBa). *European Journal of Nutrition*, 61(4), 2153–2166. https:// doi.org/10.1007/s00394-022-02798-y

Lang, A., Kuss, O., Filla, T., and Schlesinger, S. (2020). Association between Per Capita Sugar Consumption and Diabetes Prevalence Mediated by the Body Mass Index: Results of a Global Mediation Analysis. *European Journal of Nutrition*, 60(4). https://doi.org/10.1007/s00394-020-02401-2

Levine, J. A. (2011). Poverty and Obesity in the U.S. *Diabetes*, 60(11), 2667–2668. https://doi.org /10.2337/db11-1118

Li, Y., Pan, A., Wang, D. D., Liu, X., Dhana, K., Franco, O. H., Kaptoge, S., Di Angelantonio, E., Stampfer, M., Willett, W. C., and Hu, F. B. (2018). Impact of Healthy Lifestyle Factors on Life Expectancies in the US Population. *Circulation*, 138(4), 345–355. https://doi.org/10.1161 /CIRCULATIONAHA.117.032047

Lien, L., Lien, N., Heyerdahl, S., Thoresen, M., and Bjertness, E. (2006). Consumption of Soft Drinks and Hyperactivity, Mental Distress, and Conduct Problems among Adolescents in Oslo, Norway. *American Journal of Public Health*, 96(10), 1815–1820. https://doi.org/10.2105/AJPH .2004.059477

Makarem, N., Bandera, E. V., Lin, Y., Jacques, P. F., Hayes, R. B., and Parekh, N. (2018). Consumption of Sugars, Sugary Foods, and Sugary Beverages in Relation to Adiposity-Related Cancer Risk in the Framingham Offspring Cohort (1991–2013). *Cancer Prevention Research* (Philadelphia, Pa.), 11(6), 347–358. https://doi.org/10.1158/1940-6207.CAPR-17-0218

Malik, V. S., Li, Y., Pan, A., De Koning, L., Schernhammer, E., Willett, W. C., and Hu, F. B. (2019). Long-Term Consumption of Sugar-Sweetened and Artificially Sweetened Beverages and Risk of Mortality in US Adults. *Circulation*, 139(18), 2113–2125. https://doi.org/10.1161 /circulationaha.118.037401

Malik, V. S., Popkin, B. M., Bray, G. A., Després, J.-P., Willett, W. C., and Hu, F. B. (2010). Sugar-Sweetened Beverages and Risk of Metabolic Syndrome and Type 2 Diabetes: A Meta-Analysis. *Diabetes Care*, 33(11), 2477–2483. https://doi.org/10.2337/dc10-1079

Masana, M. F., Tyrovolas, S., Kolia, N., Chrysohoou, C., Skoumas, J., Haro, J. M., Tousoulis, D., Papageorgiou, C., Pitsavos, C., and Panagiotakos, D. B. (2019). Dietary Patterns and Their Association with Anxiety Symptoms among Older Adults: The ATTICA Study. *Nutrients*, 11(6), 1250. https://doi.org/10.3390/nu11061250

McAuley, K. A., Hopkins, C. M., Smith, K. J., McLay, R. T., Williams, S. M., Taylor, R. W., and Mann, J. I. (2004). Comparison of High-Fat and High-Protein Diets with a High-Carbohydrate Diet in Insulin-Resistant Obese Women. *Diabetologia*, 48(1), 8–16. https://doi.org/10.1007/s00125 -004-1603-4

References

Meng, Y., Li, S., Khan, J., Dai, Z., Li, C., Hu, X., Shen, Q., and Xue, Y. (2021). Sugar- and Artificially Sweetened Beverages Consumption Linked to Type 2 Diabetes, Cardiovascular Diseases, and All-Cause Mortality: A Systematic Review and Dose-Response Meta-Analysis of Prospective Cohort Studies. *Nutrients*, 13(8), 2636. https://doi.org/10.3390/nu13082636

Miles, F. L., Neuhouser, M. L., and Zhang, Z.-F. (2018). Concentrated Sugars and Incidence of Prostate Cancer in a Prospective Cohort. *British Journal of Nutrition*, 120(6), 703–710. https://doi .org/10.1017/s0007114518001812

Moore, J. X., Chaudhary, N., and Akinyemiju, T. (2017). Metabolic Syndrome Prevalence by Race/Ethnicity and Sex in the United States, National Health and Nutrition Examination Survey, 1988–2012. *Preventing Chronic Disease*, 14(14). https://doi.org/10.5888/pcd14.160287

Mörkl, S., Wagner-Skacel, J., Lahousen, T., Lackner, S., Holasek, S. J., Bengesser, S. A., Painold, A., Holl, A. K., and Reininghaus, E. (2018). The Role of Nutrition and the Gut-Brain Axis in Psychiatry: A Review of the Literature. *Neuropsychobiology*, 1–9. Advance online publication. https://doi.org/10.1159/000492834

National Cancer Institute. (2017). Obesity and Cancer. *National Cancer Institute*. Accessed July 31, 2022. https://www.cancer.gov/about-cancer/causes-prevention/risk/obesity/obesity-fact-sheet

National Institute of Mental Health. (2018, February). Depression. *National Institute of Mental Health*. Accessed July 31, 2022. https://www.nimh.nih.gov/health/topics/depression

———. (2021, March). Substance Use and Co-Occurring Mental Disorders. *National Institute of Mental Health*. Accessed July 31, 2022. https://www.nimh.nih.gov/health/topics/substance -use-and-mental-health

Nguyen, T. T., Ta, Q., Nguyen, T., Nguyen, T., and Giau, V. V. (2020). Type 3 Diabetes and Its Role Implications in Alzheimer's Disease. *International Journal of Molecular Sciences*, 21(9), 3165. https://doi.org/10.3390/ijms21093165

Pérez-Ara, M. Á., Gili, M., Visser, M., Penninx, B., Brouwer, I. A., Watkins, E., Owens, M., García-Toro, M., Hegerl, U., Kohls, E., Bot, M., and Roca, M. (2020). Associations of Non-Alcoholic Beverages with Major Depressive Disorder History and Depressive Symptoms Clusters in a Sample of Overweight Adults. *Nutrients*, 12(10), 3202. https://doi.org/10.3390/nu12103202

Ptacek, R., Kuzelova, H., Stefano, G. B., Raboch, J., Sadkova, T., Goetz, M., and Kream, R. M. (2014). Disruptive Patterns of Eating Behaviors and Associated Lifestyles in Males with ADHD. *Medical Science Monitor: International Medical Journal of Experimental and Clinical Research*, 20, 608–613. https://doi.org/10.12659/MSM.890495

Qin, P., Li, Q., Zhao, Y., Chen, Q., Sun, X., Liu, Y., Li, H., Wang, T., Chen, X., Zhou, Q., Guo, C., Zhang, D., Tian, G., Liu, D., Qie, R., Han, M., Huang, S., Wu, X., Li, Y., Feng, Y., and Zhang, M. (2020). Sugar and Artificially Sweetened Beverages and Risk of Obesity, Type 2 Diabetes Mellitus, Hypertension, and All-Cause Mortality: A Dose-Response Meta-Analysis of Prospective Cohort Studies. *European Journal of Epidemiology*, 35(7), 655–671. https://doi.org/10 .1007/s10654-020-00655-y

Rath, L. (n.d.). Cancer and Sugar: Is There a Link? *WebMD*. Accessed July 31, 2022. https://www .webmd.com/cancer/features/cancer-sugar-link

Rawlings, A. M., Sharrett, A. R., Albert, M. S., Coresh, J., Windham, B. G., Power, M. C., Knopman, D. S., Walker, K., Burgard, S., Mosley, T. H., Gottesman, R. F., and Selvin, E. (2019). The Association of Late-Life Diabetes Status and Hyperglycemia with Incident Mild Cognitive Impairment and Dementia: The ARIC Study. *Diabetes Care*, 42(7), 1248–1254. https://doi.org /10.2337/dc19-0120

References

Rhea, E. M., and Banks, W. A. (2019). Role of the Blood-Brain Barrier in Central Nervous System Insulin Resistance. *Frontiers in Neuroscience*, 13, 521. https://doi.org/10.3389/fnins.2019.00521

Ricciuto, L., Fulgoni, V. L., 3rd, Gaine, P. C., Scott, M. O., and DiFrancesco, L. (2021). Sources of Added Sugars Intake among the U.S. Population: Analysis by Selected Sociodemographic Factors Using the National Health and Nutrition Examination Survey 2011–18. *Frontiers in Nutrition*, 8, 687643. https://doi.org/10.3389/fnut.2021.687643

Rico-Campà, A., Martínez-González, M. A., Alvarez-Alvarez, I., Mendonça, R. D., de la Fuente-Arrillaga, C., Gómez-Donoso, C., and Bes-Rastrollo, M. (2019). Association between Consumption of Ultra-Processed Foods and All Cause Mortality: SUN Prospective Cohort Study. *BMJ (Clinical Research Ed.)*, 365, l1949. https://doi.org/10.1136/bmj.l1949

Ruby, J. G., Wright, K. M., Rand, K. A., Kermany, A., Noto, K., Curtis, D., Varner, N., Garrigan, D., Slinkov, D., Dorfman, I., Granka, J. M., Byrnes, J., Myres, N., and Ball, C. (2018). Estimates of the Heritability of Human Longevity Are Substantially Inflated due to Assortative Mating. *Genetics*, 210(3), 1109–1124. https://doi.org/10.1534/genetics.118.301613

Sanchez-Villegas, A., Zazpe, I., Santiago, S., Perez-Cornago, A., Martinez-Gonzalez, M. A., and Lahortiga-Ramos, F. (2018). Added Sugars and Sugar-Sweetened Beverage Consumption, Dietary Carbohydrate Index and Depression Risk in the Seguimiento Universidad de Navarra (SUN) Project. *The British Journal of Nutrition*, 119(2), 211–221. https://doi.org/10.1017/S0007114517003361

Satokari, R. (2020). High Intake of Sugar and the Balance between Pro- and Anti-Inflammatory Gut Bacteria. *Nutrients*, 12(5), 1348. https://doi.org/10.3390/nu12051348

Singh, G. M., Micha, R., Khatibzadeh, S., Lim, S., Ezzati, M., and Mozaffarian, D. (2015). Estimated Global, Regional, and National Disease Burdens Related to Sugar-Sweetened Beverage Consumption in 2010. *Circulation*, 132(8), 639–666. https://doi.org/10.1161/circulationaha.114.010636

Smart Label. (2022). *Kellogg's*. Accessed July 31, 2022. https://smartlabel.kelloggs.com/Product/Index/00038000143656

Srour, B., Fezeu, L. K., Kesse-Guyot, E., Allès, B., Debras, C., Druesne-Pecollo, N., Chazelas, E., Deschasaux, M., Hercberg, S., Galan, P., Monteiro, C. A., Julia, C., and Touvier, M. (2020). Ultraprocessed Food Consumption and Risk of Type 2 Diabetes Among Participants of the NutriNet-Santé Prospective Cohort. *JAMA Internal Medicine*, 180(2), 283. https://doi.org/10.1001/jamainternmed.2019.5942

Stanhope, K. L., Medici, V., Bremer, A. A., Lee, V., Lam, H. D., Nunez, M. V., Chen, G. X., Keim, N. L., and Havel, P. J. (2015). A Dose-Response Study of Consuming High-Fructose Corn Syrup–Sweetened Beverages on Lipid/Lipoprotein Risk Factors for Cardiovascular Disease in Young Adults. *The American Journal of Clinical Nutrition*, 101(6), 1144–1154. https://doi.org/10.3945/ajcn.114.100461

Te Morenga, L. A., Howatson, A. J., Jones, R. M., and Mann, J. (2014). Dietary Sugars and Cardiometabolic Risk: Systematic Review and Meta-Analyses of Randomized Controlled Trials of the Effects on Blood Pressure and Lipids. *The American Journal of Clinical Nutrition*, 100(1), 65–79. https://doi.org/10.3945/ajcn.113.081521

Thomas, D. E., and Elliott, E. J. (2010). The Use of Low-Glycaemic Index Diets in Diabetes Control. *British Journal of Nutrition*, 104(6), 797–802. https://doi.org/10.1017/s0007114510001534

Trust for America's Health. (2020). The State of Obesity 2020: Better Policies for a Healthier America. *Tfah.org*. Accessed July 31, 2022. https://www.tfah.org/report-details/state-of-obesity-2020/

References

Understanding Cardiovascular Disease: MedlinePlus Medical Encyclopedia. (2016). *Medlineplus.gov*. Accessed July 31, 2022. https://medlineplus.gov/ency/patientinstructions/000759.htm

Weinstein, G., Maillard, P., Himali, J. J., Beiser, A. S., Au, R., Wolf, P. A., Seshadri, S., and DeCarli, C. (2015). Glucose Indices Are Associated with Cognitive and Structural Brain Measures in Young Adults. *Neurology*, 84(23), 2329–2337. https://doi.org/10.1212/WNL .0000000000001655

Woo, H. D., Kim, D. W., Hong, Y. S., Kim, Y. M., Seo, J. H., Choe, B. M., Park, J. H., Kang, J. W., Yoo, J. H., Chueh, H. W., Lee, J. H., Kwak, M. J., and Kim, J. (2014). Dietary Patterns in Children with Attention Deficit/Hyperactivity Disorder (ADHD). *Nutrients*, 6(4), 1539–1553. https://doi.org/10.3390/nu6041539

World Health Organization. (2015). Guideline: Sugars Intake for Adults and Children. *www.who.int*. Accessed July 31, 2022. https://www.who.int/publications/i/item/9789241549028

———. (2020, April 1). Obesity and Overweight. *www.who.int*. Accessed July 31, 2022. https:// www.who.int/news-room/fact-sheets/detail/obesity-and-overweight

Xu, G., Strathearn, L., Liu, B., Yang, B., and Bao, W. (2018). Twenty-Year Trends in Diagnosed Attention-Deficit/Hyperactivity Disorder Among US Children and Adolescents, 1997–2016. *JAMA Network Open*, 1(4), e181471. https://doi.org/10.1001/jamanetworkopen.2018.1471

Yang, Q., Zhang, Z., Gregg, E. W., Flanders, W. D., Merritt, R., and Hu, F. B. (2014). Added Sugar Intake and Cardiovascular Diseases Mortality among US adults. *JAMA Internal Medicine*, 174(4), 516–524. https://doi.org/10.1001/jamainternmed.2013.13563

Yi, S.-Y., Steffen, L. M., Terry, J. G., Jacobs, D. R., Duprez Jr., D., Steffen, B. T., Zhou, X., Shikany, J. M., Harnack, L., and Carr, J. J. (2020). Added Sugar Intake Is Associated with Pericardial Adipose Tissue Volume. *European Journal of Preventive Cardiology*, 27(18), 2016–2023. https://doi .org/10.1177/2047487320931303

Yin, J., Zhu, Y., Malik, V., Li, X., Peng, X., Zhang, F. F., Shan, Z., and Liu, L. (2021). Intake of Sugar-Sweetened and Low-Calorie Sweetened Beverages and Risk of Cardiovascular Disease: A Meta-Analysis and Systematic Review. *Advances in Nutrition* (Bethesda, Md.), 12(1), 89–101. https://doi.org/10.1093/advances/nmaa084

CHAPTER 2

Amazon. (n.d.). Philadelphia Blueberry Cream Cheese Spread (7.5 oz Tub). *Amazon.com*. Accessed April 29, 2022. https://www.amazon.com/Philadelphia-Cream-Cheese-Spread-Blueberry/dp /B00L8CYQ3G

American Heart Association. (2021). Added Sugars. *Heart.org*. Accessed April 29, 2022. https:// www.heart.org/en/healthy-living/healthy-eating/eat-smart/sugar/added-sugars

Anton, S. D., Martin, C. K., Han, H., Coulon, S., Cefalu, W. T., Geiselman, P., and Williamson, D. A. (2010). Effects of Stevia, Aspartame, and Sucrose on Food Intake, Satiety, and Postprandial Glucose and Insulin Levels. *Appetite*, 55(1), 37–43.

Bocarsly, M. E., Powell, E. S., Avena, N. M., and Hoebel, B. G. (2010). High-Fructose Corn Syrup Causes Characteristics of Obesity in Rats: Increased Body Weight, Body Fat and Triglyceride Levels. *Pharmacology, Biochemistry, and Behavior*, 97(1), 101–106. https://doi.org/10.1016/j.pbb .2010.02.012

References

Bray, G. A., Nielsen, S. J., and Popkin, B. M. (2004). Consumption of High-Fructose Corn Syrup in Beverages May Play a Role in the Epidemic of Obesity. *The American Journal of Clinical Nutrition*, 79(4), 537–543. https://doi.org/10.1093/ajcn/79.4.537

CDC. (2021, January 27). Know Your Limit for Added Sugars. *Centers for Disease Control and Prevention.* Accessed July 31, 2022. https://www.cdc.gov/nutrition/data-statistics/added-sugars .html

Center for Food Safety and Applied Nutrition. (2018). High Fructose Corn Syrup Questions and Answers. *U.S. Food and Drug Administration.* Accessed July 31, 2022. https://www.fda.gov/food /food-additives-petitions/high-fructose-corn-syrup-questions-and-answers

Chen, H., Wang, J., Li, Z., Lam, C., Xiao, Y., Wu, Q., and Zhang, W. (2019). Consumption of Sugar-Sweetened Beverages Has a Dose-Dependent Effect on the Risk of Non-Alcoholic Fatty Liver Disease: An Updated Systematic Review and Dose-Response Meta-Analysis. *International Journal of Environmental Research and Public Health*, 16(12), 2192. https://doi.org/10 .3390/ijerph16122192

Chocolate Chip. (n.d.). *Clif Bar.* Accessed June 23, 2022. https://shop.clifbar.com/products/clif-bar -chocolate-chip

Dakhili, S., Abdolalizadeh, L., Hosseini, S. M., Shojaee-Aliabadi, S., and Mirmoghtadaie, L. (2019). Quinoa Protein: Composition, Structure and Functional Properties. *Food Chemistry*, 299, 125161. https://doi.org/10.1016/j.foodchem.2019.125161

Daniels, L. A. (1984, November 7). Coke, Pepsi to Use More Corn Syrup. *The New York Times.* Accessed July 31, 2022. https://www.nytimes.com/1984/11/07/business/coke-pepsi-to-use -more-corn-syrup.html

Davidson, T. L., Martin, A. A., Clark, K., and Swithers, S. E. (2011). Intake of High-Intensity Sweeteners Alters the Ability of Sweet Taste to Signal Caloric Consequences: Implications for the Learned Control of Energy and Body Weight Regulation. *Quarterly Journal of Experimental Psychology* (2006), 64(7), 1430–1441. https://doi.org/10.1080/17470218.2011.552729

DiGiorno Frozen Pizza. (n.d.). *Walmart.com.* Accessed June 23, 2022. https://www.walmart.com /ip/DIGIORNO-Frozen-Pizza-Frozen-Pepperoni-Pizza-27-5-oz-Rising-Crust-Pizza-27-5-oz /25826933

Dowis, K., and Banga, S. (2021). The Potential Health Benefits of the Ketogenic Diet: A Narrative Review. *Nutrients*, 13(5), 1654. https://doi.org/10.3390/nu13051654

Fowler, S. (2016). Low-Calorie Sweetener Use and Energy Balance: Results from Experimental Studies in Animals, and Large-Scale Prospective Studies in Humans. *Physiology & Behavior*, 164(Pt B), 517–523. https://doi.org/10.1016/j.physbeh.2016.04.047

George, E. S., Forsyth, A., Itsiopoulos, C., Nicoll, A. J., Ryan, M., Sood, S., Roberts, S. K., and Tierney, A. C. (2018). Practical Dietary Recommendations for the Prevention and Management of Nonalcoholic Fatty Liver Disease in Adults. *Advances in Nutrition* (Bethesda, Md.), 9(1), 30–40. https://doi.org/10.1093/advances/nmx007

Greek Whips!® Strawberry • Yoplait. (n.d.). *Yoplait.* Accessed June 23, 2022. https://www.yoplait .com/products/greek-whips-strawberry/

Green Machine. (n.d.). *Nakedjuice.com.* https://www.nakedjuice.com/our-products/machines/green -machine/

Grembecka, M. (2015). Sugar Alcohols—Their Role in the Modern World of Sweeteners: A Review. *European Food Research and Technology*, 241(1), 1–14. https://doi.org/10.1007/s00217-015-2437-7

References

Haldar, S., Egli, L., De Castro, C. A., Tay, S. L., Koh, M., Darimont, C., Mace, K., and Henry, C. J. (2020). High or Low Glycemic Index (GI) Meals at Dinner Results in Greater Postprandial Glycemia Compared with Breakfast: A Randomized Controlled Trial. *BMJ Open Diabetes Research & Care*, 8(1), e001099. https://doi.org/10.1136/bmjdrc-2019-001099

Hannou, S. A., Haslam, D. E., McKeown, N. M., and Herman, M. A. (2018). Fructose Metabolism and Metabolic Disease. *The Journal of Clinical Investigation*, 128(2), 545–555. https://doi.org/10.1172/JCI96702

Hantzidiamantis, P. J., and Lappin, S. L. (2020). Physiology, Glucose. *PubMed; StatPearls Publishing*. Accessed July 31, 2022. https://www.ncbi.nlm.nih.gov/books/NBK545201/

Hu, M., Li, M., Jiang, B., and Zhang, T. (2021). Bioproduction of D-allulose: Properties, applications, purification, and future perspectives. *Comprehensive Reviews in Food Science and Food Safety*, 20(6), 6012–6026. https://doi.org/10.1111/1541-4337.12859

Hyperglycemia Support Foundation. (n.d.). Added Sugar Repository. *Hypoglycemia.org*. Accessed June 22, 2022. https://hypoglycemia.org/added-sugar-repository/

Jensen, T., Abdelmalek, M. F., Sullivan, S., Nadeau, K. J., Green, M., Roncal, C., Nakagawa, T., Kuwabara, M., Sato, Y., Kang, D. H., Tolan, D. R., Sanchez-Lozada, L. G., Rosen, H. R., Lanaspa, M. A., Diehl, A. M., and Johnson, R. J. (2018). Fructose and Sugar: A Major Mediator of Non-Alcoholic Fatty Liver Disease. *Journal of Hepatology*, 68(5), 1063–1075. https://doi.org/10.1016/j.jhep.2018.01.019

Kellogg's® Special K® Fruit & Yogurt Cereal—SmartLabel™. (2022). *Kelloggs.com*. Accessed July 30, 2022. https://smartlabel.kelloggs.com/Product/Index/00038000482441

Lindberg, S. (2019, October 16). Nutritional Facts: Pure Maple Syrup vs. White Sugar. *LIVESTRONG.COM*. Accessed July 31, 2022. https://www.livestrong.com/article/326813 -nutritional-facts-pure-maple-syrup-vs-white-sugar/

Nabors, L. O., and Gelardi, R. C. (1986). Alternative Sweeteners. *Journal of Implied Toxicology*, 7(2), 150. https://doi.org/10.1002/jat.2550070216

McCabe, S. (2019, June 7). Brown Sugar vs. White Sugar: What's the Difference? *Healthline*. Accessed July 31, 2022. https://www.healthline.com/nutrition/brown-sugar-vs-white -sugar#production

Miller, P. E., and Perez, V. (2014). Low-Calorie Sweeteners and Body Weight and Composition: A Meta-Analysis of Randomized Controlled Trials and Prospective Cohort Studies. *The American Journal of Clinical Nutrition*, 100(3), 765–777. https://doi.org/10.3945/ajcn.113.082826

Monk Fruit. (n.d.). *Foodinsight.org*. Accessed June 23, 2022. https://foodinsight.org/wp-content /uploads/2015/08/IFIC_Monk-Fruit_Interactive.v2.pdf

National Center for Biotechnology Information. (2022). PubChem Compound Summary for CID 5988, Sucrose. Accessed June 23, 2022. https://pubchem.ncbi.nlm.nih.gov/compound /Sucrose

Neacşu, N., and Madar, A. (2014). Artificial Sweeteners versus Natural Sweeteners. *Bulletin of the Transilvania University of Braşov Series V: Economic Sciences*, 7(56), 59–64. http://rs.unitbv.ro /BU2014/Series%20V/BULETIN%20V%20PDF/08_NEACSU-MADAR%20A.pdf

Oats and Honey Granola Nature Valley. (n.d.). *Nature Valley US Headless CMS*. Accessed June 23, 2022. https://www.naturevalley.com/products/oats-honey-protein-granola

Röder, P. V., Wu, B., Liu, Y., and Han, W. (2016). Pancreatic Regulation of Glucose Homeostasis. *Experimental & Molecular Medicine*, 48(3), e219. https://doi.org/10.1038/emm.2016.6

References

Samuel, P., Ayoob, K. T., Magnuson, B. A., Wölwer-Rieck, U., Jeppesen, P. B., Rogers, P. J., Rowland, I., and Mathews, R. (2018). Stevia Leaf to Stevia Sweetener: Exploring Its Science, Benefits, and Future Potential. *The Journal of Nutrition*, 148(7), 1186S1205S. https://doi.org/10.1093/jn/nxy102

Smeets, P. A., de Graaf, C., Stafleu, A., van Osch, M. J., and van der Grond, J. (2005). Functional Magnetic Resonance Imaging of Human Hypothalamic Responses to Sweet Taste and Calories. *The American Journal of Clinical Nutrition*, 82(5), 1011–1016. https://doi.org/10.1093/ajcn/82.5.1011

Softic, S., Stanhope, K. L., Boucher, J., Divanovic, S., Lanaspa, M. A., Johnson, R. J., and Kahn, C. R. (2020). Fructose and Hepatic Insulin Resistance. *Critical Reviews in Clinical Laboratory Sciences*, 57(5), 308–322. https://doi.org/10.1080/10408363.2019.1711360

Sollid, K. (2018, August 22). Sugars: What's in a Name? *Food Insight*. Accessed July 31, 2022. https://foodinsight.org/sugars-whats-in-a-name/

———. (2020, November 20). What is Fructose? *Food Insight*. Accessed July 31, 2022. https://foodinsight.org/what-is-fructose/

———. (2020, December 23). What is Honey? *Food Insight*. Accessed July 31, 2022. https://foodinsight.org/what-is-honey/

Starbucks®. (n.d.). *Starbucks.com*. Accessed June 23, 2022. https://www.starbucks.com/menu/product/413/hot/nutrition

Stice, E., Spoor, S., Bohon, C., Veldhuizen, M. G., and Small, D. M. (2008). Relation of Reward from Food Intake and Anticipated Food Intake to Obesity: A Functional Magnetic Resonance Imaging Study. *Journal of Abnormal Psychology*, 117(4), 924–935. https://doi.org/10.1037/a0013600

Strawberry Banana BODYARMOR Sports Drinks Superior Hydration. (n.d.). *BODYARMOR*. Accessed July 31, 2022. https://www.drinkbodyarmor.com/product/strawberry-banana/

The Sugar Association. (2018). Types of Sugar. *The Sugar Association*. Accessed July 31, 2022. https://www.sugar.org/sugar/types/

Swithers, S. E. (2015). Not So Sweet Revenge: Unanticipated Consequences of High-Intensity Sweeteners. *The Behavior Analyst*, 38(1), 1–17. https://doi.org/10.1007/s40614-015-0028-3

Swithers, S. E., Martin, A. A., and Davidson, T. L. (2010). High-Intensity Sweeteners and Energy Balance. *Physiology & Behavior*, 100(1), 55–62. https://doi.org/10.1016/j.physbeh.2009.12.021

U.S. Department of Agriculture. (2019). FoodData Central. *Usda.gov*. Accessed July 31, 2022. https://fdc.nal.usda.gov/

USDA. (2020). Bagel. *Fcd.nal.usda.gov*. Accessed April 29, 2022. https://fdc.nal.usda.gov/fdc-app.html#/food-details/1100713/nutrients.

Yu, E. L., and Schwimmer, J. B. (2021). Epidemiology of Pediatric Nonalcoholic Fatty Liver Disease. *Clinical Liver Disease*, 17(3), 196–199. https://doi.org/10.1002/cld.1027

Zhang, X., Yang, S., Chen, J., and Su, Z. (2019). Unraveling the Regulation of Hepatic Gluconeogenesis. *Frontiers in Endocrinology*, 9, 802. https://doi.org/10.3389/fendo.2018.00802

CHAPTER 3

Avena, N. M., Bocarsly, M. E., Rada, P., Kim, A., and Hoebel, B. G. (2008). After Daily Bingeing on a Sucrose Solution, Food Deprivation Induces Anxiety and Accumbens Dopamine/Acetylcholine Imbalance. *Physiology & Behavior*, 94(3), 309–315. https://doi.org/10.1016/j.physbeh.2008.01.008

Avena, N. M., Long, K. A., and Hoebel, B. G. (2005). Sugar-Dependent Rats Show Enhanced Responding for Sugar after Abstinence: Evidence of a Sugar Deprivation Effect. *Physiology & Behavior*, 84(3), 359–362. https://doi.org/10.1016/j.physbeh.2004.12.016

Avena, N. M., Rada, P., and Hoebel, B. G. (2008). Evidence for Sugar Addiction: Behavioral and Neurochemical Effects of Intermittent, Excessive Sugar Intake. *Neuroscience & Biobehavioral Reviews*, 32(1), 20–39. https://doi.org/10.1016/j.neubiorev.2007.04.019

Belfort-DeAguiar, R. and Seo, D. (2018). Food Cues and Obesity: Overpowering Hormones and Energy Balance Regulation. *Current Obesity Reports*, 7(2), 122–129. https://doi.org/10.1007/s13679-018-0303-1

Boswell, R. G. and Kober, H. (2016). Food Cue Reactivity and Craving Predict Eating and Weight Gain: A Meta-Analytic Review. *Obesity Reviews: An Official Journal of the International Association for the Study of Obesity*, 17(2), 159–177. https://doi.org/10.1111/obr.12354

Colantuoni, C., Rada, P., McCarthy, J., Patten, C., Avena, N. M., Chadeayne, A., and Hoebel, B. G. (2002). Evidence That Intermittent, Excessive Sugar Intake Causes Endogenous Opioid Dependence. *Obesity Research*, 10(6), 478–488. https://doi.org/10.1038/oby.2002.66

Cravings. (2021). *The Nutrition Source*. https://www.hsph.harvard.edu/nutritionsource/cravings/

Engelmann, J. M., Versace, F., Robinson, J. D., Minnix, J. A., Lam, C. Y., Cui, Y., et al. (2012). Neural Substrates of Smoking Cue Reactivity: A Meta-Analysis of fMRI Studies. *Neuroimage*, 60(1), 252–262. https://doi.org/10.1016/j.neuroimage.2011.12.024

Galic, M. A. and Persinger, M. A. (2002). Voluminous Sucrose Consumption in Female Rats: Increased "Nippiness" during Periods of Sucrose Removal and Possible Oestrus Periodicity. *Psychological Reports*, 90(1), 58–60. https://doi.org/10.2466/pr0.2002.90.1.58

Gearhardt, A. N., Bragg, M. A., Pearl, R. L., Schvey, N. A., Roberto, C. A., and Brownell, K. D. (2012). Obesity and Public Policy. *Annual Review of Clinical Psychology*, 8, 405–430. https://doi.org/10.1146/annurev-clinpsy-032511-143129

Gearhardt, A. N., Corbin, W. R., and Brownell, K. D. (2009). Preliminary Validation of the Yale Food Addiction Scale. *Appetite*, 52(2), 430–436. https://doi.org/10.1016/j.appet.2008.12.003

———. (2016). Development of the Yale Food Addiction Scale Version 2.0. *Psychology of Addictive Behaviors: Journal of the Society of Psychologists in Addictive Behaviors*, 30(1), 113–121. https://doi.org/10.1037/adb0000136

Gearhardt, A. N., Yokum, S., Orr, P. T., Stice, E., Corbin, W. R., and Brownell, K. D. (2011). Neural Correlates of Food Addiction. *Archives of General Psychiatry*, 68(8), 808–16. https://doi.org/10.1001/archgenpsychiatry.2011.32

Harris, J. L., Bargh, J. A., and Brownell, K. D. (2009). Priming Effects of Television Food Advertising on Eating Behavior. *Health Psychology: Official Journal of the Division of Health Psychology, American Psychological Association*, 28(4), 404–413. https://doi.org/10.1037/a0014399

Hauck, C., Weiß, A., Schulte, E. M., Meule, A., and Ellrott, T. (2017). Prevalence of "Food Addiction" as Measured with the Yale Food Addiction Scale 2.0 in a Representative German Sample and Its Association with Sex, Age and Weight Categories. *Obesity Facts*, 10(1), 12–24. https://doi.org/10.1159/000456013

References

Joyner, M. A., Gearhardt, A. N., and White, M. A. (2015). Food Craving as a Mediator between Addictive-Like Eating and Problematic Eating Outcomes. *Eating Behaviors*, 19, 98–101. https://doi.org/10.1016/j.eatbeh.2015.07.005

Kharb, R., Shekhawat, L. S., Beniwal, R. P., Bhatia, T., and Deshpande, S. N. (2018). Relationship between Craving and Early Relapse in Alcohol Dependence: A Short-Term Follow-up Study. *Indian Journal of Psychological Medicine*, 40(4), 315–321. https://doi.org/10.4103/IJPSYM.IJPSYM_558_17

Kühnisch, J., Ifland, S., Tranaeus, S., and Heinrich-Weltzien, R. (2009). Comparison of Visual Inspection and Different Radiographic Methods for Dentin Caries Detection on Occlusal Surfaces. *Dentomaxillofacial Radiology*, 38(7), 452–457. https://doi.org/10.1259/dmfr/34393803

Lennerz, B. S., Alsop, D. C., Holsen, L. M., Stern, E., Rojas, R., Ebbeling, C. B., et al. (2013). Effects of Dietary Glycemic Index on Brain Regions Related to Reward and Craving in Men. *The American Journal of Clinical Nutrition*, 98(3), 641–647. https://doi.org/10.3945/ajcn.113.064113

Lim, H. K., Pae, C. U., Joo, R. H., Yoo, S. S., Choi, B. G., Kim, D. J., et al. (2005). fMRI Investigation on Cue-Induced Smoking Craving. *Journal of Psychiatric Research*, 39(3), 333–335. https://doi.org/10.1016/j.jpsychires.2004.08.004

Mangabeira, V., Garcia-Mijares, M., and Silva, M. T. (2015). Sugar Withdrawal and Differential Reinforcement of Low Rate (DRL) Performance in Rats. *Physiology & Behavior*, 139, 468–473. https://doi.org/10.1016/j.physbeh.2014.09.017

Martin, C. K., O'Neil, P. M., Tollefson, G., Greenway, F. L., and White, M. A. (2008). The Association between Food Cravings and Consumption of Specific Foods in a Laboratory Taste Test. *Appetite*, 51(2), 324–326. https://doi.org/10.1016/j.appet.2008.03.002

Massicotte, E., Deschênes, S. M., and Jackson, P. L. (2019). Food Craving Predicts the Consumption of Highly Palatable Food but Not Bland Food. *Eating and Weight Disorders—Studies on Anorexia, Bulimia and Obesity*, 24(4), 693–704. https://doi.org/10.1007/s40519-019-00706-8

Mathes, W. F., Brownley, K. A., Mo, X., and Bulik, C. M. (2009). The Biology of Binge Eating. *Appetite*, 52(3), 545–553. https://doi.org/10.1016/j.appet.2009.03.005

Mayberry, H. L., DeSalvo, H. A., Bavley, C. C., et al. (2022). Opioid and Sucrose Craving Are Accompanied by Unique Behavioral and Affective Profiles after Extended Abstinence in Male and Female Rats. *eNeuro*, 9(2), 0515–0521. https://doi.org/10.1523/ENEURO.0515-21.2022

Meule, A., Hermann, T., and Kübler, A. (2015). Food Addiction in Overweight and Obese Adolescents Seeking Weight-Loss Treatment. *European Eating Disorders Review: The Journal of the Eating Disorders Association*, 23(3), 193–198. https://doi.org/10.1002/erv.2355

Pretlow, R. A. (2011). Addiction to Highly Pleasurable Food as a Cause of the Childhood Obesity Epidemic: A Qualitative Internet Study. *Eating Disorders: The Journal of Treatment & Prevention*, 19(4), 295–307. https://doi.org/10.1080/10640266.2011.584803

Richard, A., Meule, A., Reichenberger, J., and Blechert, J. (2017). Food Cravings in Everyday Life: An EMA Study on Snack-Related Thoughts, Cravings, and Consumption. *Appetite*, 113, 215–223. https://doi.org/10.1016/j.appet.2017.02.037

Schulte, E. M., Smeal, J. K., Lewis, J., and Gearhardt, A. N. (2018). Development of the Highly Processed Food Withdrawal Scale. *Appetite*, 131, 148–154. https://doi.org/10.1016/j.appet.2018.09.013

Schulte, E. M., Yokum, S., Jahn, A., and Gearhardt, A. N. (2019). Food Cue Reactivity in Food Addiction: A Functional Magnetic Resonance Imaging Study. *Physiology & Behavior*, 208, 112574. https://doi.org/10.1016/j.physbeh.2019.112574

Stice, E., Yokum, S., Blum, K., and Bohon, C. (2010). Weight Gain Is Associated with Reduced Striatal Response to Palatable Food. *The Journal of Neuroscience: The Official Journal of the Society for Neuroscience*, 30(39), 13105–13109. https://doi.org/10.1523/JNEUROSCI.2105-10.2010

Sun, W. and Kober, H. (2020). Regulating Food Craving: From Mechanisms to Interventions. *Physiology & Behavior*, 222, 112878. https://doi.org/10.1016/j.physbeh.2020.112878

Wang, G. J., Volkow, N. D., Logan, J., Pappas, N. R., Wong, C. T., Zhu, W., et al. (2001). Brain Dopamine and Obesity. *Lancet*, 357(9253), 354–7. https://doi.org/10.1016/s0140-6736(00)03643-6

White, M. A., Whisenhunt, B. L., Williamson, D. A., Greenway, F. L., and Netemeyer, R.G. (2002). Development and Validation of the Food-Craving Inventory. *Obesity Research*, 10(2), 107–114. https://doi.org/10.1038/oby.2002.17

Wolz, I., Sauvaget, A., Granero, R., et al. (2017). Subjective Craving and Event-Related Brain Response to Olfactory and Visual Chocolate Cues in Binge-Eating and Healthy Individuals. *Scientific Reports*, 7(1). https://doi.org/10.1038/srep41736

Zimmerman, F. J. and Shimoga, S. V. (2014). The Effects of Food Advertising and Cognitive Load on Food Choices. *BMC Public Health*, 14, 342. https://doi.org/10.1186/1471-2458-14-342

CHAPTER 4

Almiron-Roig, E., Palla, L., Guest, K., Ricchiuti, C., Vint, N., Jebb, S. A., and Drewnowski, A. (2013). Factors That Determine Energy Compensation: A Systematic Review of Preload Studies. *Nutrition Reviews*, 71(7), 458–473. https://doi.org/10.1111/nure.12048

Bolthouse Farms. (2022). Strawberry Parfait. *Bolthouse Farms*. Accessed July 26, 2022. https://www.bolthouse.com/product/strawberry-parfait/

Chambers, L., McCrickerd, K., and Yeomans, M. R. (2015). Optimising Foods for Satiety. *Trends in Food Science & Technology*, 41(2), 149–160. https://doi.org/10.1016/j.tifs.2014.10.007

Chobani. (2022). Piña Colada Drink. *Chobani*. Accessed July 26, 2022. https://www.chobani.com/products/blended/drink/pina-colada/

Davis, C., Strachan, S., and Berkson, M. (2004). Sensitivity to Reward: Implications for Overeating and Overweight. *Appetite*, 42(2), 131–138. https://doi.org/10.1016/j.appet.2003.07.004

Dumanovsky, T., Nonas, C. A., Huang, C. Y., Silver, L. D., and Bassett, M. T. (2009). What People Buy from Fast-Food Restaurants: Caloric Content and Menu Item Selection, New York City 2007. *Obesity* (Silver Spring, Md.), 17(7), 1369–1374. https://doi.org/10.1038/oby.2009.90

Dunkin'. (2022). Iced Signature Latte. *Dunkin'*. Accessed July 25, 2022. https://www.dunkindonuts.com/en/menu/espresso-and-coffee/product-iced-signature-latte-id1200702

Fanelli, S., Walls, C., and Taylor, C. (2021). Skipping Breakfast Is Associated with Nutrient Gaps and Poorer Diet Quality among Adults in the United States. *Proceedings of the Nutrition Society*, 80(OCE1), E48. https://doi.org/10.1017/S0029665121000495

References

Fedewa, A. L. and Davis, M. C. (2015). How Food as a Reward Is Detrimental to Children's Health, Learning, and Behavior. *The Journal of School Health*, 85(9), 648–658. https://doi.org/10.1111/josh.12294

Fitvine Wine. (2022). Cabernet Sauvignon. *Fitvine Wine*. Accessed July 26, 2022. https://www.fitvinewine.com/products/fitvine-wine-cabernet-sauvignon

FoodSafety.gov. (2022). Cold Food Storage Chart. *FoodSafety.gov*. Accessed July 12, 2022. https://www.foodsafety.gov/food-safety-charts/cold-food-storage-charts

Galioto, R. and Spitznagel, M. B. (2016). The Effects of Breakfast and Breakfast Composition on Cognition in Adults. *Advances in Nutrition* (Bethesda, Md.), 7(3), 576S–589S. https://doi.org/10.3945/an.115.010231

Gately, M. J. Manipulation Drive in Experimentally Naïve Rhesus Monkeys [master's thesis]. Madison, WI: University of Wisconsin, 1950.

Harlow, H. F., Harlow, M. K., and Meyer, D. R. (1950). Learning Motivated by a Manipulation Drive. *Journal of Experimental Psychology*, 40(2), 228–234. https://doi.org/10.1037/h0056906

Harvard T.H. Chan School of Public Health. (2019, October 16). Sugary Drinks. *The Nutrition Source*. Accessed January 30, 2022. https://www.hsph.harvard.edu/nutritionsource/healthy-drinks/sugary-drinks/

Lu, J., Xiong, S., Arora, N., and Dubé, L. (2015). Using Food as Reinforcer to Shape Children's Non-Food Behavior: The Adverse Nutritional Effect Doubly Moderated by Reward Sensitivity and Gender. *Eating Behaviors*, 19, 94–97. https://doi.org/10.1016/j.eatbeh.2015.07.003

Malek, A. M., Newman, J. C., Hunt, K. J., Jack, M. M., and Marriott, B. P. (2019). Dietary Sources of Sugars and Calories. *Nutrition Today*, 54(6), 296–304. https://doi.org/10.1097/NT.0000000000000378

Malik, V. S., Schulze, M. B., and Hu, F. B. (2006). Intake of Sugar-Sweetened Beverages and Weight Gain: A Systematic Review. *The American Journal of Clinical Nutrition*, 84(2), 274–288. https://doi.org/10.1093/ajcn/84.1.274

Monster. (2022). Monster Energy Green Original. *HEB*. Accessed July 26, 2022. https://www.heb.com/product-detail/monster-energy-green-original-16-oz-cans/690258

Naked. (2022). Fruit Smoothie Strawberry Banana. *Naked*. Accessed July 26, 2022. https://www.nakedjuice.com/our-products/core/strawberry-banana/

Nielsen, S. J., Kit, B. K., Fakhouri, T., and Ogden, C. L. (2012). Calories Consumed from Alcoholic Beverages by U.S. Adults, 2007–2010. *NCHS Data Brief*, 2012 (110), 1–8. Accessed January 31, 2022. https://medlineplus.gov/ency/patientinstructions/000886.htm

Ocean Spray. (2022). 100% Juice Cranberry. *Ocean Spray*. Accessed July 26, 2022. https://www.oceanspray.com/Products/Juices/By-Type/100-Percent-Juice/100-Percent-Juice-Cranberry

Paccino, D. (2022). Breakfast Statistics 2022: What's the USA's Favorite Breakfast? *Kitchen Infinity*. Accessed July 11, 2022. https://kitcheninfinity.com/breakfast-statistics/

Paddon-Jones, D., Westman, E., Mattes, R. D., Wolfe, R. R., Astrup, A., and Westerterp-Plantenga, M. (2008). Protein, Weight Management, and Satiety. *The American Journal of Clinical Nutrition*, 87(5), 1558S–1561S. https://doi.org/10.1093/ajcn/87.5.1558S

Pepsico. (2022, July 20). Mountain Dew. *Pepsico Beverage Facts*. Accessed July 26, 2022. https://www.pepsicobeveragefacts.com/Home/product?formula=44316*01*01-10&form=RTD&size=20

References

————. (2022, July 20). Rockstar Original. *Pepsico Beverage Facts.* Accessed July 26, 2022. https://www.pepsicobeveragefacts.com/Home/Product?formula=BACX513&form=RTD&size=16

Razzoli, M., Pearson, C., Crow, S., and Bartolomucci, A. (2017). Stress, Overeating, and Obesity: Insights from Human Studies and Preclinical Models. *Neuroscience & Biobehavioral Reviews,* 76, 154–162. https://doi.org/10.1016/j.neubiorev.2017.01.026

Redbull. (2022). Redbull Energy Drink Ingredients. *Redbull.* Accessed July 26, 2022. https://www.redbull.com/us-en/energydrink/red-bull-energy-drink-ingredients-list

Remy, E., Issanchou, S., Chabanet, C., Boggio, V., and Nicklaus, S. (2015). Impact of Adiposity, Age, Sex and Maternal Feeding Practices on Eating in the Absence of Hunger and Caloric Compensation in Preschool Children. *International Journal of Obesity* (2005), 39(6), 925–930. https://doi.org/10.1038/ijo.2015.30

Seagram's. (2022). Seagram's Ginger Ale. *Seagram's.* Accessed July 26, 2022. https://www.seagramsgingerale.com/products/ginger-ale

Sievert, K., Hussain, S. M., Page, M. J., Wang, Y., Hughes, H. J., Malek, M., and Cicuttini, F. M. (2019). Effect of Breakfast on Weight and Energy Intake: Systematic Review and Meta-Analysis of Randomised Controlled Trials. *BMJ* (Clinical Research Ed.), 364, l42. https://doi.org/10.1136/bmj.l42

Smith, K. S. and Graybiel, A. M. (2016). Habit Formation. *Dialogues in Clinical Neuroscience,* 18(1), 33–43. https://doi.org/10.31887/DCNS.2016.18.1/ksmith

Smoothie King. (2022). Nutrition Information: Pure Recharge Strawberry. *Smoothie King.* Accessed July 26, 2022. https://www.smoothieking.com/menu/smoothies/nutrition/feel-energized-blend

Snapple. (2022). Peach Tea. *Snapple.* Accessed July 26, 2022. https://www.snapple.com/products/filter/tea/snapple-peach-tea

Starbucks. (2022). Iced Caffè Mocha. *Starbucks.* Accessed July 25, 2022. https://www.starbucks.com/menu/product/408/iced

Stookey, J. D., Constant, F., Gardner, C. D., and Popkin, B. M. (2007). Replacing Sweetened Caloric Beverages with Drinking Water Is Associated with Lower Energy Intake. *Obesity* (Silver Spring, Md.), 15(12), 3013–3022. https://doi.org/10.1038/oby.2007.359

Target. (2022). Almond Breeze Vanilla Almond Milk—0.5 gal. *Target.* Accessed July 26, 2022. https://www.target.com/p/almond-breeze-vanilla-almond-milk-0-5gal/-/A-13752452

Tropical Smoothie Café. (2022). Health and Nutrition Guide: Mango Madness. *Tropical Smoothie Café.* Accessed July 26, 2022. https://d38zwb0vf9f6v5.cloudfront.net/wp-content/uploads/2022/06/01110642/Tropical-Smoothie-Cafe-Nutrition-Guide-June-2022-1.pdf

Tropicana. (2022). Original (No Pulp). *Tropicana.* Accessed July 26, 2022. https://www.tropicana.com/products/pure-premium/original-no-pulp/

USDA. (2020). Nutrition Bar (Clif Bar). *fdc.nal.usda.gov.* Accessed March 9, 2022. https://fdc.nal.usda.gov/fdc-app.html#/food-details/1101260/nutrients

————. (2022). Almonds, Lightly Salted. *fdc.nal.usda.gov.* Accessed March 8, 2022. https://fdc.nal.usda.gov/fdc-app.html#/food-details/1100510/nutrients

————. (2022). Cheese, Cheddar. *fdc.nal.usda.gov.* Accessed March 8, 2022. https://fdc.nal.usda.gov/fdc-app.html#/food-details/328637/nutrients

References

————. (2022). Chicken Breast, Grilled without Sauce, Skin Not Eaten. *fdc.nal.usda.gov.* Accessed March 8, 2022. https://fdc.nal.usda.gov/fdc-app.html#/food-details/1098457/nutrients

————. (2022). Peach, Raw. *fdc.nal.usda.gov.* Accessed March 8, 2022. https://fdc.nal.usda.gov/fdc-app.html#/food-details/1102677/nutrients

————. (2022). Salmon, Baked or Broiled, Made with Cooking Spray. *fdc.nal.usda.gov.* Accessed March 9, 2022. https://fdc.nal.usda.gov/fdc-app.html#/food-details/1098966/nutrients

Vieira, E. F. and Souza, S. (2022). Formulation Strategies for Improving the Stability and Bioavailability of Vitamin D-Fortified Beverages: A Review. *Foods* (Basel, Switzerland), 11(6), 847. https://doi.org/10.3390/foods11060847

Welch's. (2022). 100% White Grape Juice. *Welch's.* Accessed July 26, 2022. https://www.welchs.com/juices/100-percent/white-grape

Zhang, K., Dong, R., Hu, X., Ren, C., and Li, Y. (2021). Oat-Based Foods: Chemical Constituents, Glycemic Index, and the Effect of Processing. *Foods*, 10(6), 1304. https://doi.org/10.3390/foods10061304

CHAPTER 5

Batiha, G. E., Beshbishy, A. M., Ikram, M., Mulla, Z. S., El-Hack, M., Taha, A. E., Algammal, A. M., and Elewa, Y. (2020). The Pharmacological Activity, Biochemical Properties, and Pharmacokinetics of the Major Natural Polyphenolic Flavonoid: Quercetin. *Foods* (Basel, Switzerland), 9(3), 374. https://doi.org/10.3390/foods9030374

Botezatu, N. (2017). Relative Sweetness and Nutrients of Fruits. *Medium.* Accessed February 2, 2022. https://medium.com/@nelly.botezatu/relative-sweetness-and-nutrients-of-fruits-d70169483733

Dhillon, J., Craig, B. A., Leidy, H. J., Amankwaah, A. F., Osei-Boadi Anguah, K., Jacobs, A., Jones, B. L., Jones, J. B., Keeler, C. L., Keller, C. E., McCrory, M. A., Rivera, R. L., Slebodnik, M., Mattes, R. D., and Tucker, R. M. (2016). The Effects of Increased Protein Intake on Fullness: A Meta-Analysis and Its Limitations. *Journal of the Academy of Nutrition and Dietetics*, 116(6), 968–983. https://doi.org/10.1016/j.jand.2016.01.003

DiNicolantonio, J. J., O'Keefe, J. H., and Wilson, W. L. (2018). Sugar Addiction: Is It Real? A Narrative Review. *British Journal of Sports Medicine*, 52(14), 910–913. https://doi.org/10.1136/bjsports-2017-097971

Eggersdorfer, M. and Wyss, A. (2018). Carotenoids in Human Nutrition and Health. *Archives of Biochemistry and Biophysics*, 652, 18–26. https://doi.org/10.1016/j.abb.2018.06.001

Harvard. (2022). Protein. *hsph.harvard.edu.* Accessed February 25, 2022. https://www.hsph.harvard.edu/nutritionsource/what-should-you-eat/protein

Igwe, E. O. and Charlton, K. E. (2016). A Systematic Review on the Health Effects of Plums (*Prunus domestica* and *Prunus salicina*). *Phytotherapy Research: PTR*, 30(5), 701–731. https://doi.org/10.1002/ptr.5581

Imamura, F., Micha, R., Wu, J. H., de Oliveira Otto, M. C., Otite, F. O., Abioye, A. I., and Mozaffarian, D. (2016). Effects of Saturated Fat, Polyunsaturated Fat, Monounsaturated Fat, and Carbohydrate on Glucose-Insulin Homeostasis: A Systematic Review and Meta-Analysis of Randomised Controlled Feeding Trials. *PLoS Medicine*, 13(7), e1002087. https://doi.org/10.1371/journal.pmed.1002087

Jukanti, A., Gaur, P., Gowda, C., and Chibbar, R. (2012). Nutritional Quality and Health Benefits of Chickpea (Cicer arietinum L.): A Review. *British Journal of Nutrition*, 108(S1), S11–S26. https://doi.org/10.1017/S0007114512000797

Koikeda, T., Tokudome, Y., Okayasu, M., et al. (2017). Effects of Peach (Prunus persica)-Derived Glucosylceramide on the Human Skin. *Current Medicinal Chemistry*, 17(1), 56. https://doi.org/10.2174/1871522217666170906155435

Koutsos, A., Tuohy, K. M., and Lovegrove, J. A. (2015). Apples and Cardiovascular Health—Is the Gut Microbiota a Core Consideration? *Nutrients*, 7(6), 3959–3998. https://doi.org/10.3390/nu7063959

Kulczyński, B., Kobus-Cisowska, J., Taczanowski, M., Kmiecik, D., and Gramza-Michałowska, A. (2019). The Chemical Composition and Nutritional Value of Chia Seeds—Current State of Knowledge. *Nutrients*, 11(6), 1242. https://doi.org/10.3390/nu11061242

Lima, M., Ares, G., and Deliza, R. (2019). Comparison of Two Sugar Reduction Strategies with Children: Case Study with Grape Nectars. *Food Quality and Preference*, 71, 163–167. https://doi.org/10.1016/j.foodqual.2018.07.002

NIH. (2022). Omega-3 Fatty Acids. *ods.od.nih.gov*. Accessed February 25, 2022. https://ods.od.nih.gov/factsheets/Omega3FattyAcids-HealthProfessional/

Nutrition Data. (2022). Pineapple, Raw, All Varieties. Nutrition Facts & Calories. *nutritiondata.self.com*. Accessed February 2, 2022. https://nutritiondata.self.com/facts/fruits-and-fruit-juices/2019/2

Pandey, K. B. and Rizvi, S. I. (2009). Plant Polyphenols as Dietary Antioxidants in Human Health and Disease. *Oxidative Medicine and Cellular Longevity*, 2(5), 270–278. https://doi.org/10.4161/oxim.2.5.9498

Pap, N., Fidelis, M., Azevedo, L., Carmo, M.A., Wang, D., Mocan, A., Pereira, E.P., Xavier-Santos, D., Sant'Ana, A.S., Yang, B., and Granato, D. (2021). Berry Polyphenols and Human Health: Evidence of Antioxidant, Anti-Inflammatory, Microbiota Modulation, and Cell-Protecting Effects. *Current Opinion in Food Science*, 42, 167–186. https://doi.org/10.1016/j.cofs.2021.06.003

Pavan, R., Jain, S., Shraddha, and Kumar, A. (2012). Properties and Therapeutic Application of Bromelain: A Review. *Biotechnology Research International*, 2012, 976203. https://doi.org/10.1155/2012/976203

Phillips, W. (2014). Coding for Malnutrition in the Adult Patient: What the Physician Needs to Know. *Nutritional Issues in Gastroenterology*, 133, 56–63. https://med.virginia.edu/ginutrition/wp-content/uploads/sites/199/2014/06/Parrish-Sept-14.pdf

Rasmussen, H. M. and Johnson, E. J. (2013). Nutrients for the Aging Eye. *Clinical Interventions in Aging*, 8, 741–748. https://doi.org/10.2147/CIA.S45399

Reiland, H. and Slavin, J. (2015). Systematic Review of Pears and Health. *Nutrition Today*, 50(6), 301–305. https://doi.org/10.1097/NT.0000000000000112

Roberts, J. E. and Dennison, J. (2015). The Photobiology of Lutein and Zeaxanthin in the Eye. *Journal of Ophthalmology*, 2015, 687173. https://doi.org/10.1155/2015/687173

Rock, C. L., Zunshine, E., Nguyen, H. T., Perez, A. O., Zoumas, C., Pakiz, B., and White, M. M. (2020). Effects of Pistachio Consumption in a Behavioral Weight Loss Intervention on Weight Change, Cardiometabolic Factors, and Dietary Intake. *Nutrients*, 12(7), 2155. https://doi.org/10.3390/nu12072155

References

Salehi, B., Fokou, P., Sharifi-Rad, M., Zucca, P., Pezzani, R., Martins, N., and Sharifi-Rad, J. (2019). The Therapeutic Potential of Naringenin: A Review of Clinical Trials. *Pharmaceuticals* (Basel, Switzerland), 12(1), 11. https://doi.org/10.3390/ph12010011

Schlörmann, W. and Glei, M. (2017). Potential Health Benefits of β-Glucan from Barley and Oat. *Ernahrungs Umschau*, 64(10): 145–149. https://www.ernaehrungs-umschau.de/fileadmin /Ernaehrungs-Umschau/pdfs/pdf_2017/10_17/EU10_2017_WuF_Glei_englisch.pdf

USDA. (2019). Apricots, Raw. *fdc.nal.usda.gov*. Accessed February 2, 2022. https://fdc.nal.usda.gov /fdc-app.html#/food-details/171697/nutrients

———. (2019). Cherries, Sweet, Raw. *fdc.nal.usda.gov*. Accessed February 1, 2022. https://fdc.nal .usda.gov/fdc-app.html#/food-details/171719/nutrients

———. (2019). Oranges, Raw, Navels. *fdc.nal.usda.gov*. Accessed February 2, 2022. https://fdc.nal .usda.gov/fdc-app.html#/food-details/746771/nutrients

———. (2019). Peaches, Yellow, Raw. *fdc.nal.usda.gov*. Accessed February 2, 2022. https://fdc.nal .usda.gov/fdc-app.html#/food-details/325430/nutrients

———. (2019). Pears, Raw, Bartlett. *fdc.nal.usda.gov*. Accessed February 2, 2022. https://fdc.nal .usda.gov/fdc-app.html#/food-details/746773/nutrients

———. (2020). Apple, Raw. *fdc.nal.usda.gov*. Accessed February 1, 2022. https://fdc.nal.usda.gov /fdc-app.html#/food-details/1102644/nutrients

———. (2020). Banana, Raw. *fdc.nal.usda.gov*. Accessed February 1, 2022. https://fdc.nal.usda.gov /fdc-app.html#/food-details/1102653/nutrients

———. (2020). Chicken Breast, Grilled without Sauce, Skin Not Eaten. *fdc.nal.usda.gov*. Accessed February 25, 2022. https://fdc.nal.usda.gov/fdc-app.html#/food-details/1098457/ nutrients

———. (2020). Egg Omelet or Scrambled Egg, No Added Fat. *fdc.nal.usda.gov*. Accessed February 25, 2022. https://fdc.nal.usda.gov/fdc-app.html#/food-details/1100240/nutrients

———. (2020). Kiwi Fruit, Raw. *fdc.nal.usda.gov*. Accessed February 2, 2022. https://fdc.nal.usda .gov/fdc-app.html#/food-details/1102667/nutrients

———. (2020). Mango, Raw. *fdc.nal.usda.gov*. Accessed February 1, 2022. https://fdc.nal.usda.gov /fdc-app.html#/food-details/1102670/nutrients

———. (2020). Salmon, Baked or Broiled, No Added Fat. *fdc.nal.usda.gov*. Accessed February 25, 2022. https://fdc.nal.usda.gov/fdc-app.html#/food-details/1098965/nutrients

———. (2022). Protein Foods. *myplate.gov*. Accessed February 25, 2022. https://www.myplate.gov /eat-healthy/protein-foods

Valls, R. M., Pedret, A., Calderón-Pérez, L., Llauradó, E., Pla-Pagà, L., Companys, J., Moragas, A., Martín-Luján, F., Ortega, Y., Giralt, M., Romeu, M., Rubió, L., Mayneris-Perxachs, J., Canela, N., Puiggrós, F., Caimari, A., Del Bas, J. M., Arola, L., and Solà, R. (2021). Effects of Hesperidin in Orange Juice on Blood and Pulse Pressures in Mildly Hypertensive Individuals: A Randomized Controlled Trial (Citrus Study). *European Journal of Nutrition*, 60(3), 1277–1288. https://doi.org/10.1007/s00394-020-02279-0

Westwater, M. L., Fletcher, P. C., and Ziauddeen, H. (2016). Sugar Addiction: The State of the Science. *European Journal of Nutrition*, 55(Suppl 2), 55–69. https://doi.org/10.1007/s00394-016 -1229-6

References

Wilkinson-Smith, V., Dellschaft, N., Ansell, J., Hoad, C., Marciani, L., Gowland, P., and Spiller, R. (2019). Mechanisms Underlying Effects of Kiwifruit on Intestinal Function Shown by MRI in Healthy Volunteers. *Alimentary Pharmacology & Therapeutics*, 49(6), 759–768. https://doi.org /10.1111/apt.15127

Zaman, S. A. and Sarbini, S. R. (2016). The Potential of Resistant Starch as a Prebiotic. *Critical Reviews in Biotechnology*, 36(3), 578–584. https://doi.org/10.3109/07388551.2014.993590

Zeinalian, R., Farhangi, M. A., Shariat, A. et al. The Effects of Spirulina Platensis on Anthropometric Indices, Appetite, Lipid Profile and Serum Vascular Endothelial Growth Factor (VEGF) in Obese Individuals: A Randomized Double Blinded Placebo Controlled Trial. *BMC Complementary and Alternative Medicine*, 17, 225 (2017). https://doi.org/10.1186/s12906-017-1670-y

Zhu, L., Huang, Y., Edirisinghe, I., Park, E., and Burton-Freeman, B. (2019). Using the Avocado to Test the Satiety Effects of a Fat-Fiber Combination in Place of Carbohydrate Energy in a Breakfast Meal in Overweight and Obese Men and Women: A Randomized Clinical Trial. *Nutrients*, 11(5), 952. https://doi.org/10.3390/nu11050952

CHAPTER 6

Carbonneau, E., Lamarche, B., Robitaille, J., Provencher, V., Desroches, S., Vohl, M. C., Bégin, C., Bélanger, M., Couillard, C., Pelletier, L., Bouchard, L., Houle, J., Langlois, M. F., Corneau, L., and Lemieux, S. (2019). Social Support, but Not Perceived Food Environment, Is Associated with Diet Quality in French-Speaking Canadians from the PREDISE Study. *Nutrients*, 11(12), 3030. https://doi.org/10.3390/nu11123030

Chung, A., Vieira, D., Donley, T., Tan, N., Jean-Louis, G., Kiely Gouley, K., and Seixas, A. (2021). Adolescent Peer Influence on Eating Behaviors via Social Media: Scoping Review. *Journal of Medical Internet Research*, 23(6), e19697. https://doi.org/10.2196/19697

Cunningham, S. A., Vaquera, E., Maturo, C. C., and Narayan, K. M. (2012). Is There Evidence That Friends Influence Body Weight? A Systematic Review of Empirical Research. *Social Science & Medicine* (1982), 75(7), 1175–1183. https://doi.org/10.1016/j.socscimed.2012.05.024

Dohle, S., Hartmann, C., and Keller, C. (2014). Physical Activity as a Moderator of the Association between Emotional Eating and BMI: Evidence from the Swiss Food Panel. *Psychology & Health*, 29(9), 1062–1080. https://doi.org/10.1080/08870446.2014.909042

Folkvord, F., Roes, E., and Bevelander, K. (2020). Promoting Healthy Foods in the New Digital Era on Instagram: An Experimental Study on the Effect of a Popular Real versus Fictitious Fit Influencer on Brand Attitude and Purchase Intentions. *BMC Public Health*, 20(1), 1677. https:// doi.org/10.1186/s12889-020-09779-y

Janis, I. (1991). Groupthink. In E. Griffin (Ed.) *A First Look at Communication Theory*, 235–246. New York: McGrawHill. http://williamwolff.org/wp-content/uploads/2016/01/griffin-groupthink -challenger.pdf

Katterman, S. N., Kleinman, B. M., Hood, M. M., Nackers, L. M., and Corsica, J. A. (2014). Mindfulness Meditation as an Intervention for Binge Eating, Emotional Eating, and Weight Loss: A Systematic Review. *Eating Behaviors*, 15(2), 197–204. https://doi.org/10.1016/j.eatbeh .2014.01.005

Lawlor, E. R., Hughes, C. A., Duschinsky, R., Pountain, G. D., Hill, A. J., Griffin, S. J., and Ahern, A. L. (2020). Cognitive and Behavioural Strategies Employed to Overcome "Lapses" and Prevent "Relapse" among Weight-Loss Maintainers and Regainers: A Qualitative Study. *Clinical Obesity*, 10(5), e12395. https://doi.org/10.1111/cob.12395

Leow, S., Jackson, B., Alderson, J. A., Guelfi, K. J., and Dimmock, J. A. (2018). A Role for Exercise in Attenuating Unhealthy Food Consumption in Response to Stress. *Nutrients*, 10(2), 176. https://doi.org/10.3390/nu10020176

Mills, S., Brown, H., Wrieden, W., White, M., and Adams, J. (2017). Frequency of Eating Home Cooked Meals and Potential Benefits for Diet and Health: Cross-Sectional Analysis of a Population-Based Cohort Study. *The International Journal of Behavioral Nutrition and Physical Activity*, 14(1), 109. https://doi.org/10.1186/s12966-017-0567-y

Murphy, G., Corcoran, C., Tatlow-Golden, M., Boyland, E., and Rooney, B. (2020). See, Like, Share, Remember: Adolescents' Responses to Unhealthy-, Healthy- and Non-Food Advertising in Social Media. *International Journal of Environmental Research and Public Health*, 17(7), 2181. https://doi.org/10.3390/ijerph17072181

Popkin, B. M. and Ng, S. W. (2022). The Nutrition Transition to a Stage of High Obesity and Noncommunicable Disease Prevalence Dominated by Ultra-Processed Foods Is Not Inevitable. *Obesity Reviews: An Official Journal of the International Association for the Study of Obesity*, 23(1), e13366. https://doi.org/10.1111/obr.13366

Rounsefell, K., Gibson, S., McLean, S., Blair, M., Molenaar, A., Brennan, L., Truby, H., and McCaffrey, T. A. (2020). Social Media, Body Image and Food Choices in Healthy Young Adults: A Mixed Methods Systematic Review. *Nutrition & Dietetics: The Journal of the Dietitians Association of Australia*, 77(1), 19–40. https://doi.org/10.1111/1747-0080.12581

Rowbotham, S., Astell-Burt, T., Barakat, T., and Hawe, P. (2020). 30+ Years of Media Analysis of Relevance to Chronic Disease: A Scoping Review. *BMC Public Health*, 20(1), 364. https://doi.org/10.1186/s12889-020-8365-x

Sacks, G. and Looi, E. (2020). The Advertising Policies of Major Social Media Platforms Overlook the Imperative to Restrict the Exposure of Children and Adolescents to the Promotion of Unhealthy Foods and Beverages. *International Journal of Environmental Research and Public Health*, 17(11), 4172. https://doi.org/10.3390/ijerph17114172

Sharpe, H., Schober, I., Treasure, J., and Schmidt, U. (2014). The Role of High-Quality Friendships in Female Adolescents' Eating Pathology and Body Dissatisfaction. *Eating and Weight Disorders: EWD*, 19(2), 159–168. https://doi.org/10.1007/s40519-014-0113-8

Stults-Kolehmainen, M. A. and Sinha, R. (2014). The Effects of Stress on Physical Activity and Exercise. *Sports Medicine* (Auckland, N.Z.), 44(1), 81–121. https://doi.org/10.1007/s40279-013-0090-5

Turnwald, B. P., Anderson, K. G., Markus, H. R., and Crum, A. J. (2022). Nutritional Analysis of Foods and Beverages Posted in Social Media Accounts of Highly Followed Celebrities. *JAMA Network Open*, 5(1), e2143087. https://doi.org/10.1001/jamanetworkopen.2021.43087

Turnwald, B. P., Handley-Miner, I. J., Samuels, N. A., Markus, H. R., and Crum, A. J. (2021). Nutritional Analysis of Foods and Beverages Depicted in Top-Grossing US Movies, 1994–2018. *JAMA Internal Medicine*, 181(1), 61–70. https://doi.org/10.1001/jamainternmed.2020.5421

Versace, F., Frank, D. W., Stevens, E. M., Deweese, M. M., Guindani, M., and Schembre, S. M. (2019). The Reality of "Food Porn": Larger Brain Responses to Food-Related Cues than to Erotic Images Predict Cue-Induced Eating. *Psychophysiology*, 56(4): e13309. doi: 10.1111/psyp.13309

Yoshikawa, A., Smith, M. L., Lee, S., Towne, S. D., and Ory, M. G. (2021). The Role of Improved Social Support for Healthy Eating in a Lifestyle Intervention. *Texercise Select. Public Health Nutrition*, 24(1), 146–156. https://doi.org/10.1017/S1368980020002700

CONCLUSION

Dickson, J. M., Moberly, N. J., Preece, D., Dodd, A., and Huntley, C. D. (2021). Self-Regulatory Goal Motivational Processes in Sustained New Year Resolution Pursuit and Mental Wellbeing. *International Journal of Environmental Research and Public Health*, 18(6), 3084. https://doi.org/10.3390/ijerph18063084

Johnson, F. and Wardle, J. (2011). The Association between Weight Loss and Engagement with a Web-Based Food and Exercise Diary in a Commercial Weight Loss Programme: A Retrospective Analysis. *The International Journal of Behavioral Nutrition and Physical Activity*, 8, 83. https://doi.org/10.1186/1479-5868-8-83

Palascha, A., van Kleef, E., and van Trijp, H. C. (2015). How Does Thinking in Black and White Terms Relate to Eating Behavior and Weight Regain? *Journal of Health Psychology*, 20(5), 638–648. https://doi.org/10.1177/1359105315573440

Pi-Sunyer, X. (2009). The Medical Risks of Obesity. *Postgraduate Medicine*, 121(6), 21–33. https://doi.org/10.3810/pgm.2009.11.2074

Ricciuto, L., Fulgoni, V. L., 3rd, Gaine, P. C., Scott, M. O., and DiFrancesco, L. (2021). Sources of Added Sugars Intake Among the U.S. Population: Analysis by Selected Sociodemographic Factors Using the National Health and Nutrition Examination Survey 2011–18. *Frontiers in Nutrition*, 8, 687643. https://doi.org/10.3389/fnut.2021.687643

APPENDIX

Added Sugar Repository. Hypoglycemia Support Foundation. (n.d.). Retrieved May 7, 2022, from https://hypoglycemia.org/added-sugar-repository/

ACKNOWLEDGMENTS

There are many people whom I must thank for accompanying me on this journey. Professionally, I am forever grateful to all of my colleagues, collaborators, and students, too many to name, that I have been fortunate enough to work with and learn from over the years. My PhD mentor, Bart Hoebel, was one of my best friends, and I am so grateful to have worked with him and learned from him. Many of the studies described in this book arose out of our lab meetings, working lunches at our favorite place, Nassau Sushi/ Bagel, and discussions at conferences. Even though he died several years ago, he continues to have a huge impact on my career and life, and I am forever grateful to have been able to have him as a friend. I would also like to thank Mark Gold, who is another amazing mentor, teacher, and friend, as well as Pedro Rada, who taught me so much about neuroscience and research, and who also got me hooked on good coffee.

I would also like to thank my group of friends and colleagues who are active in the diet and mental health world. Each of you brings a much-needed voice to the conversation, and I am grateful for your inspiring work. Thank you to my friend Daniel Amen, for not only being a leader in the field of psychiatry and brain health, but also for writing the foreword. Also, thanks to Rob Lustig, Michael Goran, and Ashley Gearhardt for all your important work in this field, as well as your friendship. I am so fortunate to have been able to work alongside so many amazing and inspiring researchers over the years—too many names to list here. But I am extremely grateful for all of you.

This book would not have been possible without my amazing team of research assistants and students. Special thanks to Chloe Rosenblatt, Keally Haushalter, Julia Simkus, Paige Kerstetter, Amanda Laezza, Kaylee Hough, Ella Morgan, and Kristen Criscitelli. Thanks to Casey Elsass, who did an incredible job editing the recipes and helping to make them as delicious as possible. Also, thank you to my literary agent, Linda Konner. Knowing that I have your guidance and support makes the whole process of writing a book easier. I would also like to thank my wonderful editor at Union Square & Co., Jessica Firger, as well as the editorial director, Amanda Englander. Thank you for believing in this book (and in me!). Thanks also to the rest of the team at Union Square & Co. who worked so hard to make *Sugarless* the best it could be.

Last but never least, I want to thank my amazing friends and family. Without their support and encouragement, I would be completely lost. My husband, Eamon, is an unrelenting supporter of my work, passions, and inability to sit in idle for too long. My daughters Stella and Viv are the lights of my life and my fuel. I love you all.

INDEX

Index

Index

Index

Sandwiches
  Chickpea-Avocado
    Sandwich, 235–36
  low-carb ideas for, 141
Satiety
  biological factors, 64–65
  feeling of, 118
  from high fiber foods,
    65, 149
  from high protein foods,
    65, 150, 164–66, 177
  lack of, from beverages,
    118–20
  signaled by GLP-1, 71
Sauces
  Italian, hidden sugars
    in, 144
  Sugarless BBQ Sauce,
    250–51
Seafood
  Baked Salmon Sushi Rolls
    with Cilantro-Lime
    Rice, 232–34
  protein in, 165
Self-monitoring, 188, 193
Setbacks, managing,
  186–93
Side dishes, list of recipes,
  215
Sleep, 161, 185–86
Smoothie bowls, 109
Smoothies, 126–27
Snack bars, 59–60
Snacks
  healthy choices for,
    148–52
  list of recipes, 215
SnackWell's®, xvi
Social media, 193–95
Social pressure
  food in TV and movies,
    196
  food porn, 195
  from friends and family,
    196–201
  from social media, 193–95
  when eating out, 200–201
Soft drinks and sodas,
  122–23
Sorbitol, 68

Soups
  added sugar in, 141
  Coconut Avocado Lime
    Soup, 228–29
  Creamy Tomato and
    Roasted Red Pepper
    Soup with Grilled
    Halloumi, 226–27
Spirulina, 177–78
Sports drinks, 64
Stevia, 66
Strawberries
  Strawberry Shortcake
    Parfaits, 255–56
  Whole-Fruit Frozen
    Rocket Pops, 262–63
Stress
  beneficial, 111–12, 180
  effect on appetite, 181
  leading to overeating,
    12–13
  managing, tips for,
    183–86
  negative effects of, 112–13
  primary appraisal of, 181
  secondary appraisal of,
    181–82
Substance abuse, 74. *See also*
  Addiction
Substance use disorder, 77, 78
Sucrose, 53
Sugar. *See also* Added sugar;
  Sugar addiction
  brown, about, 52
  consumption statistics, 6
  correlation with chronic
    diseases, 17–35
  cravings for, xvii, 87,
    89–91
  evaluating intake of,
    105–10
  giving up completely,
    40–41
  long-term damage from,
    xxi–xxii, 11
  modern mindset towards,
    6
  other names for, 48–50,
    269–73
  primitive urge to eat, 7

pro-inflammatory nature
  of, 23
unrefined, 52, 57–58
Sugar addiction
  origin of term, xix
  quiz for, 280
  reinforced by food cues,
    95–98
  research studies on,
    xx–xxi, 79–81, 93–95
  withdrawal from, 84–86,
    93–94, 157–63
Sugar addiction, breaking
  admitting your addiction,
    103–5
  cutting out sweetened
    drinks, 118–33
  evaluating your sugar
    intake, 105–10
  ground rules for, 100–102
  identifying triggers,
    110–17
  rethinking breakfast,
    134–40
  rethinking dinner, 140–45
  rethinking lunch, 145–48
  rethinking snacks, 148–52
Sugar alcohols, 67–69
Sugar-sweetened drinks
  and breastfeeding, 25
  categories of, 122–31
  coffee, 122
  correlation with cancer,
    23–24
  correlation with
    depression, 29
  correlation with
    premature death,
    33–34
  drinkable yogurts, 127–28
  energy drinks, 123–25
  how they lead to weight
    gain, 118–20
  juices, 125–26
  milks, 128–31
  during pregnancy, 25
  smoothies, 126–27
  soft drinks and sodas,
    122–23
  sports drinks, 64

ABOUT THE AUTHOR

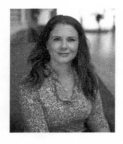

DR. NICOLE AVENA is an associate professor of neuroscience at Mount Sinai School of Medicine in New York City, and a visiting professor of health psychology at Princeton University. She is a research neuroscientist and expert in the fields of nutrition, diet, and addiction, with a special focus on nutrition throughout the life span and health psychology. She has done groundbreaking work developing models to characterize food addiction and develop new treatments for overeating and obesity. She also has conducted pioneering studies on the dangers of excess sugar intake. Her research achievements have been honored by awards from several groups, including the New York Academy of Sciences, the American Psychological Association, and the National Institute on Drug Abuse. In addition to over a hundred peer-reviewed scholarly publications, Dr. Avena has written several books, including *Why Diets Fail, What to Eat When You're Pregnant, What to Feed Your Baby and Toddler,* and *What to Eat When You Want to Get Pregnant.* She frequently appears as a science expert in the media, including regular appearances on *The Dr. Oz Show, Good Day New York,* and *The Doctors,* as well as many other news programs. Her work has been featured in *Time, Time for Kids, Bloomberg Businessweek,* the *New York Times,* and many other media outlets. Dr. Avena is a member of the Penguin Random House Speakers Bureau. Her TED-Ed Health Talk, "How Sugar Affects Your Brain," is among one of the most watched, with over 15 million views and counting. She lives in Princeton, New Jersey, with her husband, daughters, and their dog, Monty.